Happy Birthday
Ross

Love your lovely
godmother who has your
spiritual welfare
at heart xxx

Happiness
NOW

written and illustrated by
Andrew Matthews

Seashell Publishers
AUSTRALIA

Happiness NOW
Copyright © 2005 by Andrew Matthews
and Seashell Publishers

Published by:
Seashell Publishers,
PO Box 325, Trinity Beach,
Queensland, Australia, 4879.

Fax: (within Australia) 07 4057 6966
Fax: (from outside Australia) 61 7 4057 6966
Email: info@seashell.com.au
Visit our website: www.seashell.com.au

Layout and design by Twocan and Seashell Publishers
Printed by C.O.S. Printers Pte Ltd, Singapore

ISBN 978 097 57 6427 5

First published July 2005
1st reprint August 2005
2nd reprint August 2005
3rd reprint September 2005
4th reprint October 2006
5th reprint June 2007
6th reprint May 2008
7th reprint October 2009

Also by the same author:
"Being Happy!"
"Making Friends"
"Follow Your Heart"
"Happiness in a Nutshell"
"Being a Happy Teen"

To Julie:

To my precious wife and publisher – again, thank you!

Thank you for your brilliance in managing our publishing company.

Thank you for the endless long days and late nights you spend on the phone with the other side of the world, making things happen. With your energy, passion and courage, you do things that no one else could ever do!

Thank you for your wisdom and guidance.

Thank you for putting your brilliant career on hold to take these books to the world.

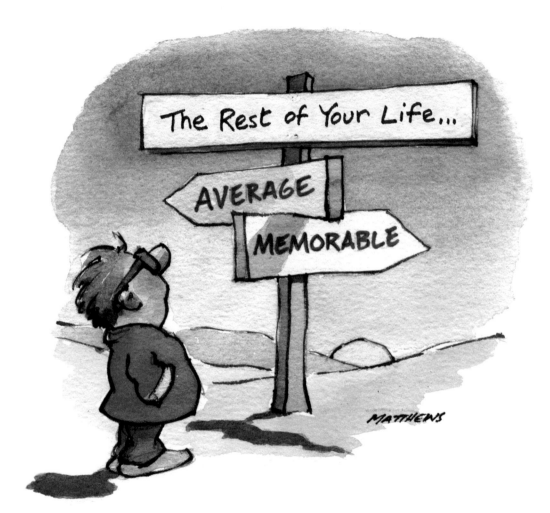

Contents

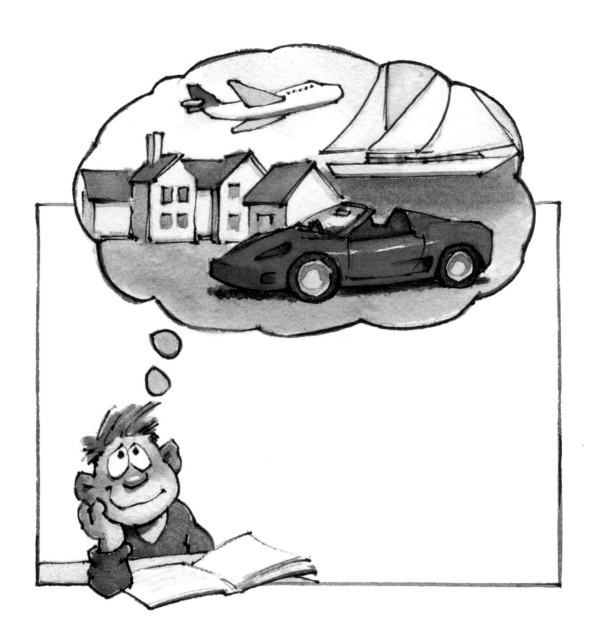

Isn't it strange? Everyone wants happiness, but where do we study it?

We are born. We go to school.

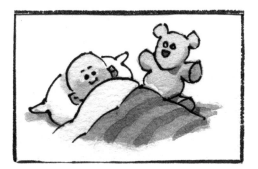 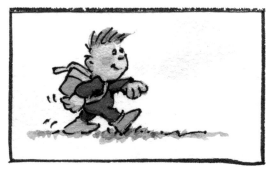

We study mathematics. We learn about haemoglobin and the Himalayas. But we never study happiness.

I used to ask myself, "Why are some people always happy?"

I wondered, "Are happy people smarter than the rest of us? Or are happy people just too silly to realise that they should be miserable?" More about that later …

When I was a kid, I used to dream about the future.

When I finally got to the future, I was often disappointed.

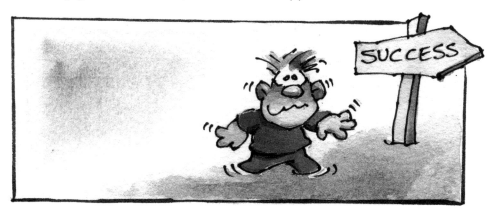

I discovered that LIFE IS HARDER THAN IT LOOKS!

I wanted to know:
"How come other people live fascinating lives?"
"How come other people are happier than me?"

I read books. I attended lectures and seminars.

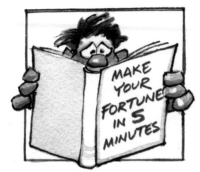 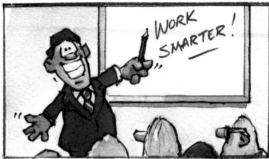

I tried walking on fire.

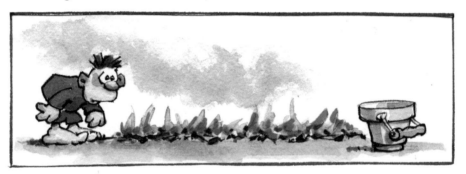

I read about the great philosophers. I figured that they could teach me about happiness ...

I came across a group of ancient Greek philosophers called the Skeptics. They said that "You can only have real peace of mind if you don't believe anything". But how can you believe that?

I read about Socrates – and a fellow called Gorgias. Gorgias said:
a) nothing really exists, therefore
b) if something did exist, you wouldn't know it, therefore
c) you don't exist!
But how can you use that information?

Imagine ... you get pulled over by a traffic cop, who says,
"Give me one reason why I shouldn't book you for speeding."
And you tell him, "You don't exist!"

I noticed two things about philosophers:
a) most of them weren't very happy, and
b) lots of them were mathematicians!

"Everyday Philosophy"

Here's what I have come to believe.

There are two kinds of philosophy – the academic kind, and the everyday, personal kind.

It is your everyday, personal philosophy that really counts.

Your everyday philosophy is what you believe about everyday stuff – about work, money, worry, failure, friendship, family, the future.

Everyday philosophy is what we use to explain life's ups and downs:
it is the foundation on which we build our life.

It's like when people say ...
"Everything happens for a reason", or
"Disasters are opportunities", or
"All men are bastards!"
It's personal!

Our personal philosophy is the lens through which we view every problem and every opportunity.

Often, it is the reason that we give ourselves to persist – or quit.

People who live happily are not necessarily the smartest or the richest or the most talented. But they have a personal philosophy that serves them well.

Happy people seem to share certain philosophies on life.

This book is a summary of the strategies of happy, effective people.

Some of these ideas will already be familiar to you. Sometimes we don't need new information – we just need to be reminded!

And a cartoon can help us to remember the message.

If you have suffered serious personal tragedy or trauma, then this book may not be enough, but it can help with your everyday challenges.

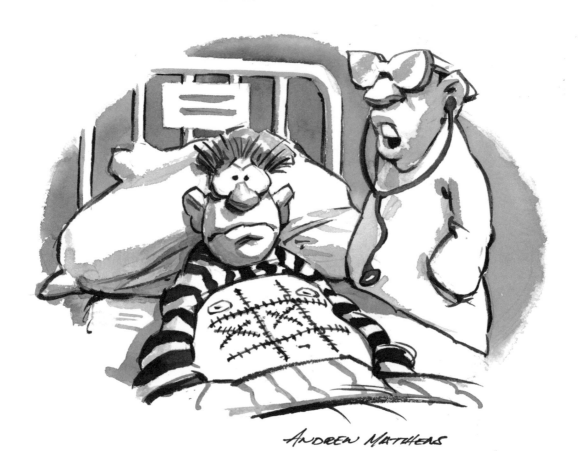

"One more operation –
we haven't beaten this thing yet."

When Things Get Tough

Happiness Myths

Kick the Worry Habit!

Character

Why?

Mental Fitness

Laughter

When Things Are Beyond Your Control

Rage!

"Where am I going?"

Patience

Isn't It Amazing?

Happiness

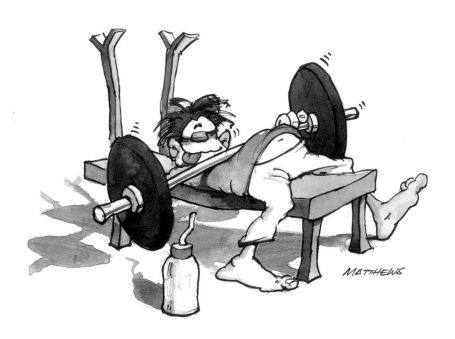

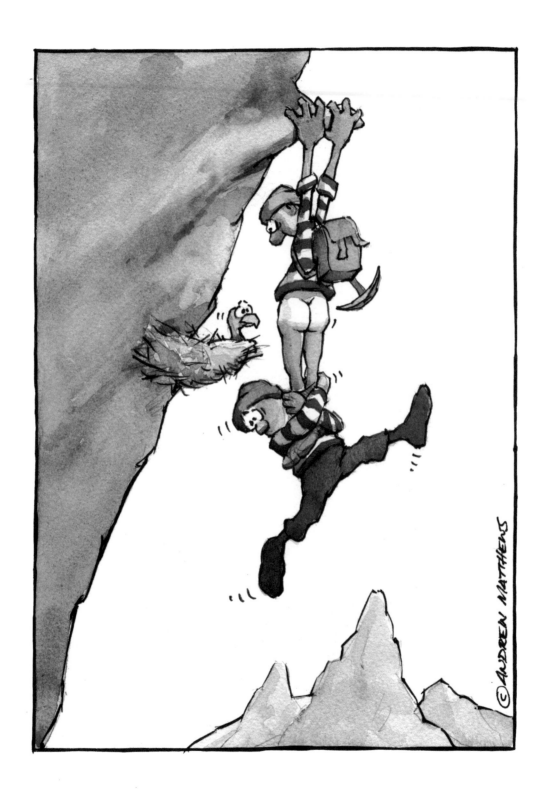

When Life Gets Tough

How do you survive when life gets tough?
How do you hang on when you are grieving, lonely or broke?

You can only tackle your problems as you would climb a mountain ...

If you go rock climbing - and you get stuck on a ledge - you suddenly focus on the present moment!

You forget about the future. All your effort goes into your next step.
Then your next step. Inch by inch.

Eventually you claw your way out.

The same strategy works for everyday life.

When things seem desperate, you fix your focus on the present moment.

You tackle one problem at a time. You take a step. You get a little confidence ... and take another step, and another.

Eventually you find that the worst is over.

If you were to worry about
    a) everything you need to do in the next month, or
    b) everything that could go wrong in the next year,
    you could go nuts!

But you can handle one day at a time.

And whenever 24 hours is too tough, bite off five minutes at a time.

IN A NUTSHELL

All you can do is give your best effort until bedtime.
Let tomorrow take care of itself.

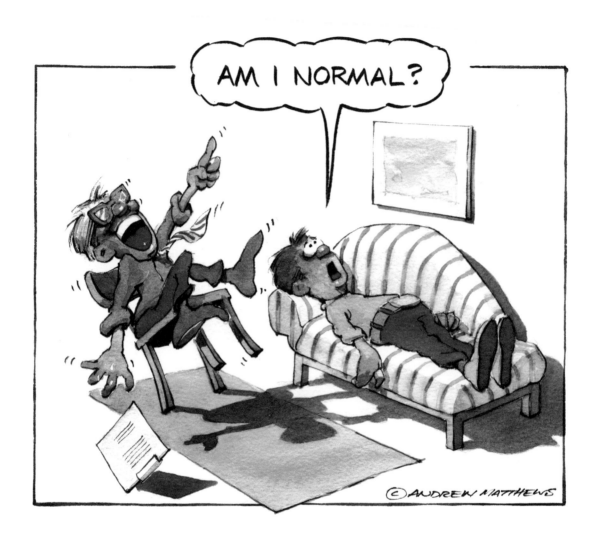

Happiness Myths

In the 1990s researcher Ronald Inglehart published the results of a massive "happiness survey" involving 170,000 people from 16 countries.

The participants were asked questions like, "How happy are you?" and "Are you satisfied with your life?"

Inglehart was interested to see whether our age affects our happiness. So he analysed the data by age group, 15 to 24 years old, 25 to 34 years old, 35 to 44 years and so on.

So who do you think were the most miserable? The teens? The mid-lifers? And who do you think were the happiest?

Here are the results –

15-24 years	81% satisfied with life
25-34 years	80% satisfied with life
35-44 years	80% satisfied with life
45-54 years	79% satisfied with life
55-64 years	79% satisfied with life
65 years and over.	81% satisfied with life

The results for each age group were almost identical!

In different research, Arizona State University psychologists William Stock and Morris Okun reached exactly the same conclusion. They assessed the results of over 100 psychological studies and boiled them down to this – that age has no more than a 1 percent impact on happiness!

Despite all the myths, and despite all the talk of "troubled teens" and "mid-life crises", age has almost no bearing on your happiness!

IN A NUTSHELL
It's not about your age, it's about your attitude.

SOURCES:
Data from 169,776 people reported by Robert Inglehart, Culture Shift in an Advanced Industrial Society (Princeton: Princeton University Press, 1990).
David G. Myers, The Pursuit of Happiness, Harper Collins Publishers 1992.

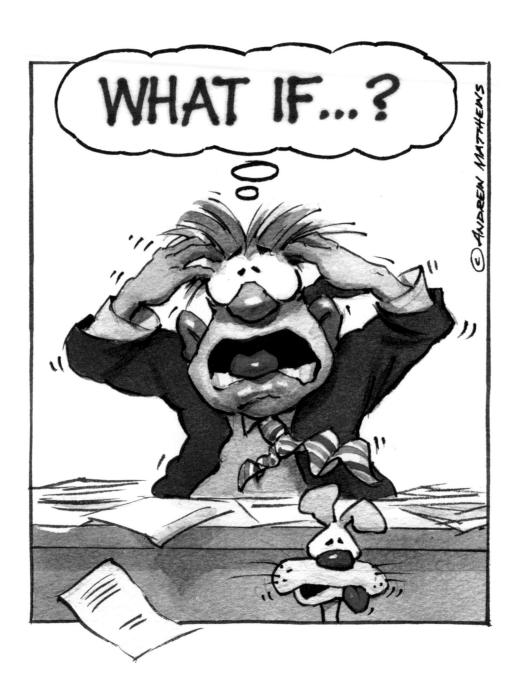

Kick the Worry Habit!

Most of us worry.
We worry about our jobs, our children ... and what the neighbours think!

Some people will even tell you, "You SHOULD worry!"

But worrying is WORSE THAN USELESS!
Firstly, it attracts misfortune.
Secondly, it is bad for your health!

So what should you do about worry? Postpone it!
Take action FIRST and postpone worry indefinitely.
That's what effective people do.

Whenever you want to worry, ask yourself,
"What is the problem right this second?"

Guess what you'll find ... unless you are in a life-threatening situation, you don't have a problem!

Of course, disasters do happen. Illness happens. Financial crises happen. That's no reason to live life like a frightened rabbit.

When crises come, you can deal with them MOMENT BY MOMENT.
It's only when your mind drifts into the future that it crushes you.
And your mind *will* want to drag you into the future!

Stay in the present! Do whatever you can do today –
and leave worry out of it.

Look at your life. Has there ever been a situation that you didn't survive? There hasn't!

You can handle the present. It's just the future that gives you trouble!

IN A NUTSHELL
When it comes to worry, procrastinate!
When someone asks, "Aren't you worried about that?" tell them,
"I've been meaning to worry about it – but I haven't got around to it!"

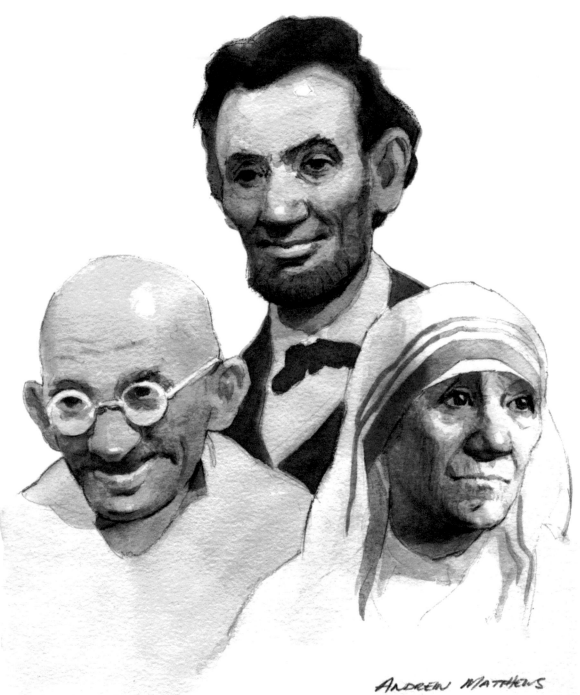

ANDREW MATTHEWS

Character

Did you ever look in the mirror and say,
"I wish I had a different face ... body ... nose?"

Did you ever look at your life and say,
"How come other people are so talented and brilliant?
How can I feel good about me?"

Most of us have these thoughts!

But here's the crunch ...

Talent and beauty are very useful – but there are plenty of talented and beautiful people around whom we don't necessarily admire. And some of them are a pain in the neck!

Many of history's most admired people – like Abraham Lincoln, Mother Theresa and Mahatma Ghandi – were neither beautiful nor especially gifted.

The qualities most of us value above all others are HONESTY, COURAGE, PERSISTENCE, GENEROSITY and HUMILITY.

Take a look at this list and you'll find something interesting.
You aren't BORN with these qualities.
You DEVELOP them.
Anyone can have them.
If you really want, you can have them!

If you want self-respect, and respect from others, you don't have to be a genius or a super-model.

You simply work at developing your own honesty, determination, generosity, humility and courage.

It is called "character".

IN A NUTSHELL
How you feel about you is in your hands.

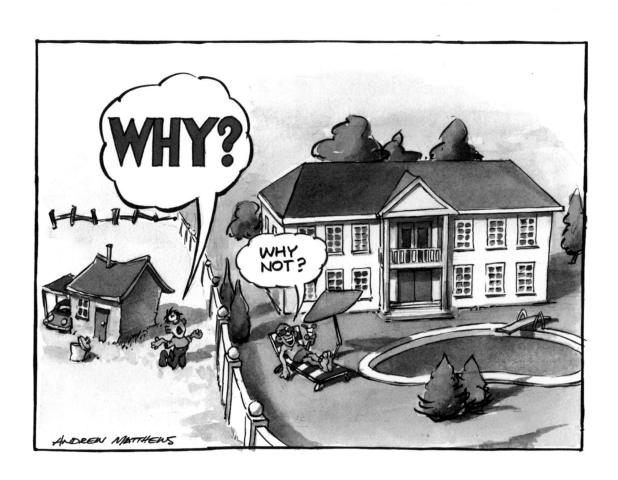

"Why?"

My friend John Foppe was born with no arms.
But John never asks the question,
"WHY do I have no arms?"
The question he asks is,
"WHAT can I do with my feet?"

Having watched John eat with chopsticks, I'd say,
"Almost anything!"

When tragedy strikes, or when we lose everything, or when a lover walks out on us, the question we usually ask is "WHY?"
"WHY me?"
"WHY now?"
"WHY did she leave me for a loser?"

Asking "WHY?" questions can send us crazy.
Often, there is no answer to "WHY?"
Or it doesn't matter why!

Effective people ask "WHAT?" questions ...
"WHAT am I going to do about it?"
"WHAT do I learn from this?"

When the situation is really desperate, they ask,
"WHAT can I do, just in the next 24 hours, to make things better?"

IN A NUTSHELL

The happiest people don't bother about whether life is fair.
They just make the most of what they have.

And is life "fair"? Probably not. But it doesn't matter why!

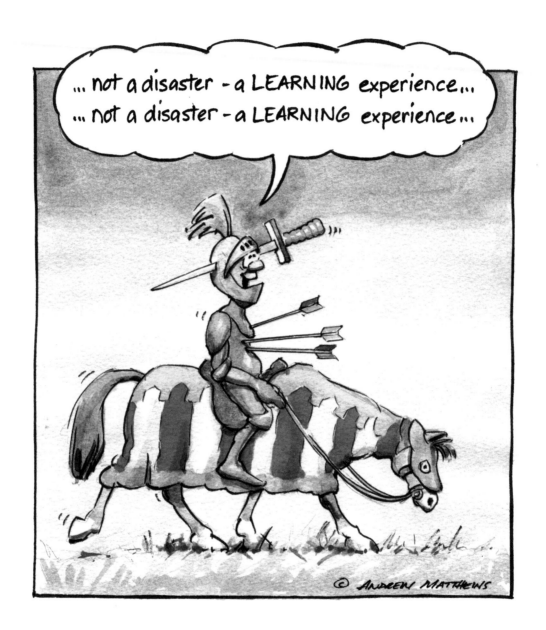

Mental Fitness

You'll notice something about most happy people ...
they have overcome serious set-backs.

Happy people sometimes go broke, get sick, get sacked – or get dumped!
Like everyone, happy people have their problems.
But they have the mental strength to focus on solutions.
They have developed "mental fitness".

Mental fitness is like physical fitness.

You strengthen your MUSCLES with exercise.
You run uphill.
Gradually you get stronger.

It is the same with your thinking.
You strengthen your MIND by facing problems.

STRUGGLE builds STRENGTH.

You don't get strong by hiding under the bed.
You meet life head on.
You take some risks.
You fail and bounce back.

Day by day you gain confidence.
Gradually you build a positive attitude.

When life gets rough, remind yourself:
"This is making me mentally fit. I must be getting happier!"

IN A NUTSHELL

It is not necessarily an easy life that makes you happy.
Usually it's the opposite!

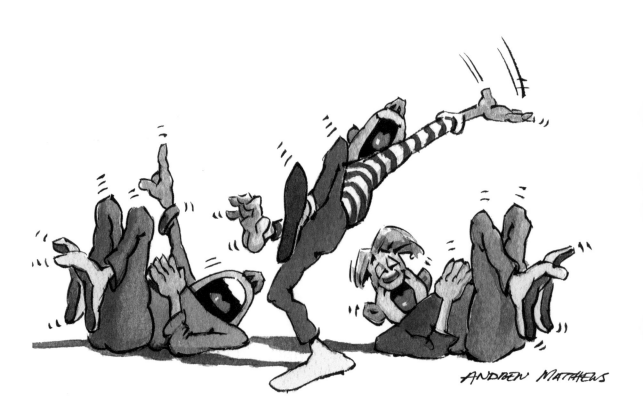

Laughter

Did you ever bump your head or break a wrist while you were clowning around with friends? What did you notice?

While you are LAUGHING, it is hard to feel PAIN!

All kinds of wonderful things happen when you laugh ...

- Your lung capacity expands, improving respiration and oxygen consumption
- Your immune system is activated – so you can better fight infection. Your body releases more of the protective T cells that fight virus and cancer cells
- Endorphins – your body's natural painkillers – are released into your brain, decreasing stress.

Laughter not only reduces physical pain. It reduces mental pain!

When we laugh, we naturally feel more hopeful and optimistic.
When we laugh, we say to ourselves – and to the world –
"I REFUSE TO SUFFER!"

Laughter helps us survive grief and disappointment.

There's a funny side to almost every situation. We just have to look for it.

What else helps? When we stop trying to be perfect!

When we stop trying to be perfect, we can laugh at ourselves – so we laugh much more often.

IN A NUTSHELL
Life is not that serious. We should take humour more seriously!

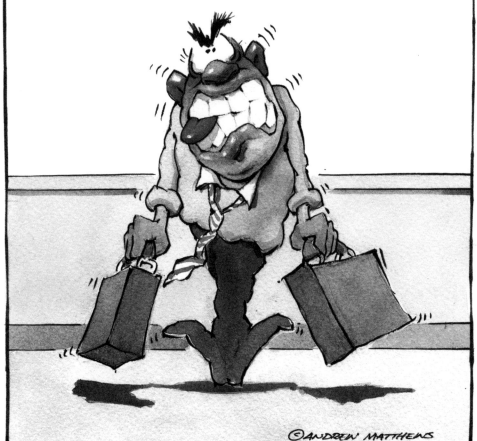

When Things Are Beyond Your Control

Here's a recipe for permanent misery ...
   a) Decide how you think the world SHOULD be.
   b) Make rules for how everyone SHOULD behave.

Then, when the world doesn't obey your rules, get angry!
That's what miserable people do!

Let's say you expect that:
Friends SHOULD return favours.
People SHOULD appreciate you.
Planes SHOULD arrive on time.
Everyone SHOULD be honest.
Your husband SHOULD remember your birthday.

These expectations may sound reasonable. But often, these things
won't happen! So you end up frustrated and disappointed.

There's a better strategy. Don't have so many demands.
Instead, have preferences!

For things that are beyond your control, tell yourself:
"I WOULD PREFER "A", BUT IF "B" HAPPENS, IT'S OK TOO!"

This is really a game that you play in your head.
But if you make the game a habit, you have more peace of mind ...

You prefer that people are polite ...
but when they are rude, it doesn't ruin your day.
You prefer sunshine ... but rain is ok!
In other words, you practise flexibility.

To become happier, we need to either a) change the world, or
b) change our thinking. It is easier to change our thinking!

IN A NUTSHELL
It's not what happens to you that determines your happiness.
It's how you think about what happens to you.

ROAD rage

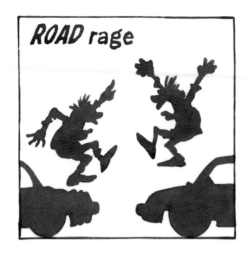

AIR rage

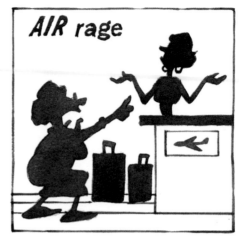

FOOD rage

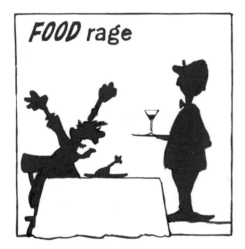

FAN rage

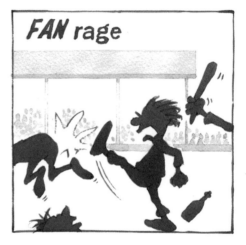

PHONE rage

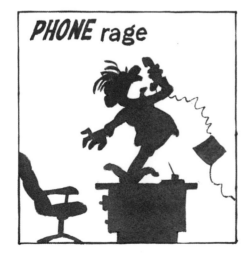

OUT rage

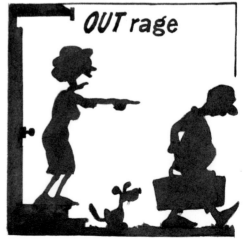

Rage!

These days getting angry is all the rage. We've got road rage, restaurant rage, supermarket rage, phone rage, hospital rage ... it's outrageous! Here's what's interesting about rage ...

It's usually not what happens to us that makes us angry.
It's when we expect one thing to happen but something else happens ...

EXAMPLE:
You are driving on the highway and you decide to change lanes.
You EXPECT the guy in the next lane to make room for you – but he doesn't!
You EXPECT him to be considerate – but he isn't. So you get mad.

The problem here is not the other driver – it is your expectation that he should be nice! Expectation sets us up for disappointment and anger.

Most people won't think like you and your plans will often go wrong. So the fewer expectations you have about the world – and even the weather –
the better life gets!

Three more tips for keeping your cool:

1. HUMILITY HELPS! Angry people tend to believe that a) they are more important than everyone else, and b) that they are always right. When they don't get what they want, they get angry! Relax a little. Allow for others to sometimes get what they want.

2. DECIDE WHAT IS REALLY IMPORTANT in your life, say, on a scale from one to ten. You might rank having enough food to eat at 9 out of 10.
   You might rank having a job at 7 out of 10, idiot drivers at 2 out of 10, and slow elevators at zero. When you have things in perspective, you don't get upset over details.

3. ACCEPT WHAT IS. Angry people love to argue with reality! They say things like, "It shouldn't be raining!" or "Thieves shouldn't steal!" It is a waste of energy. When you argue with reality, reality wins!

IN A NUTSHELL

There are six and a half billion other people on planet earth. For them to sometimes get what they want, we sometimes need to go without.
That's no reason to shout at people and beat them up.

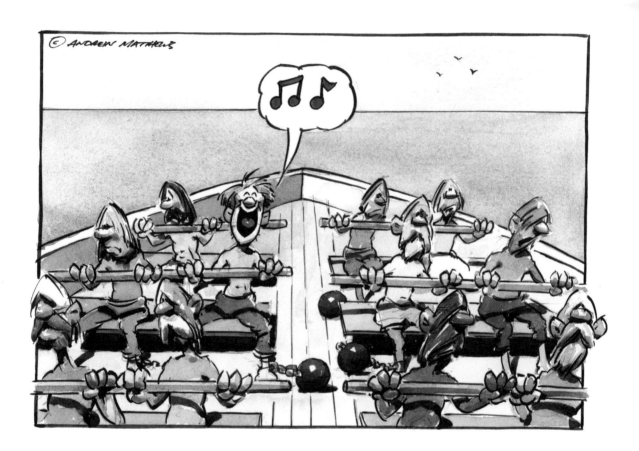

"Where am I going?"

Did you ever ask yourself: "What am I doing in this stupid job?"
Do you ever feel like you are stuck?

If you feel frustrated or unhappy at work – whether you're a chicken plucker or a brain surgeon – your best strategy is ... GIVE IT ALL YOU'VE GOT.

Why?
- You feel better about yourself
- You develop your skills
- You develop a reputation
- Sometime, someone will notice you and offer you a better position, or
- You'll one day get the confidence to go do your own thing.

Fred says, "If I had a great job, I would really work hard – but I've got this lousy job so I just sleep all day!" No, Fred!

When we continually give our best, life naturally leads us toward new opportunities. Sometimes it takes a while, but it happens.

One more thing ... opportunities, job offers – and romance – usually arrive when we least expect them.

Great opportunities and life-changing relationships mostly happen in the most unlikely situations.

It's life's way of reminding us to give respect to everyone we meet.

It's also life's way of reminding us to keep an open mind!

Successful people tell themselves, "If I make the most of this opportunity, I'll get a bigger one".

IN A NUTSHELL

Life rewards effort, not excuses.

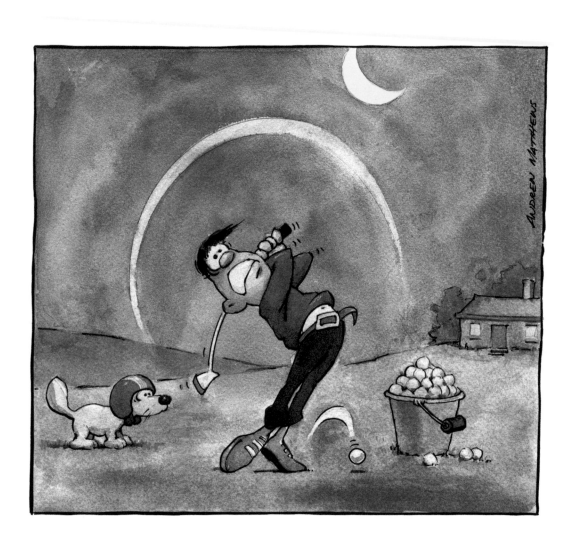

Patience

A woman approached the great violinist Fritz Kreisler after one of his concerts. She said, "Mr Kreisler, I would give my life to play as you play!"
He turned and smiled and said, "I DID!"

If you want to be really good at something, you might need to spend your whole life practising – or ten years practising – or at least six months!

A hundred years ago, most people understood this.

Nowadays, people want instant results!

For whatever you want to do, here's a strategy ... practise every day, but don't expect to see progress every day!

If you are:
- getting your body fit
- learning a language
- refining your golf swing
- taking singing lessons
- learning a new sport, beginning a hobby, starting a new career, give yourself enough time.

Get a daily plan, stick with it *AND* allow yourself time to improve.

You might see little progress in a month. Give it six months of effort – or a year of effort – THEN assess your improvement.

Most people quit too soon!

IN A NUTSHELL

To be successful, this is what you need - in order of importance:
1. patience and persistence
2. talent.

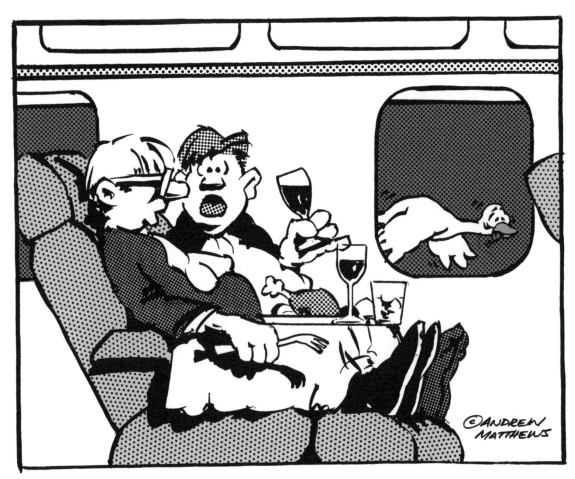

"All this flying can really tire you out!"

Isn't it Amazing?

Fred boards a jumbo jet in Bangkok at 11.30pm. The jet seats 420 people and it weighs as much as a small apartment block.

For the next 14 hours Fred travels at over 800 kilometres an hour. Less than a foot from his nose the air temperature is minus 55 degrees Celsius and the wind is blowing at hurricane strength.

Meanwhile the crew serves him dinner – steak from Argentina, wine from Australia, butter from Ireland, cheese from New Zealand, coffee from Columbia.

At the press of a button blankets and pillows are delivered.

Fred buys duty free watches for the kids without even leaving his seat. During dessert he watches the latest Hollywood movies.

He takes a nap. For breakfast, it's croissants and fruit.

And all this in economy class!

At 5.00 am London time, in the middle of a hailstorm with 10 metres visibility, he touches down on the other side of the world – two minutes ahead of schedule.

Fred's wife collects him at the airport ... "How was your flight?"
And Fred says, "Nothing special!"
Nothing special? It's amazing! We take so much for granted!

We live in an extraordinary world. We are so fortunate to eat food we didn't have to grow and fish we didn't catch, to drive in cars that we didn't have to invent across bridges we didn't have to build.

IN A NUTSHELL
Any flight that lands safely is a good flight!

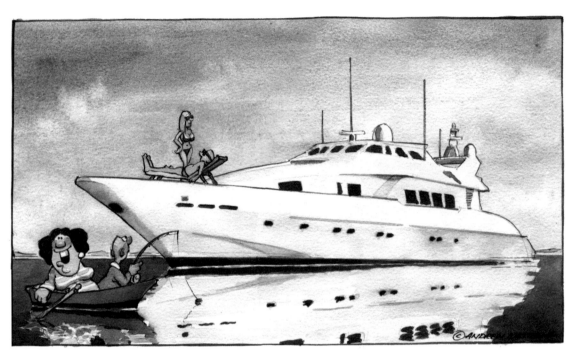

*"They're not happy.
They just **think** they're happy."*

Happiness

You don't wait for life to get easier.
You make the choice to be happy first.

I remember waiting for my life to get easier. I thought, "When I have less problems, I'll be happy!"

Then I noticed something fascinating. The happiest people I knew had more problems than I did!

Maybe you have noticed the same thing – that people who seem to get the most out of life have often had it tough. They have lost loved ones, they've gone broke, they've suffered serious illness – and most likely, they still have big problems!

But they are happy because at some point they decided "happy" is the only way to live.

Happiness doesn't just happen to you, like some "accident". It is something you choose.

Recently I had a conversation on Cleveland radio with a lady called Rena.

Rena told me, "I just got divorced, I am currently being sued, my house just burned down and now my doctors tell me that my cancer has returned for the third time." But she said, "You know, amongst all this, I am happy!"

If you wake up saying, "I hope I have a good day, and then I'll be happy", you never will be.

IN A NUTSHELL

You don't find happiness in the *absence* of problems.
You find it *in spite* of your problems!

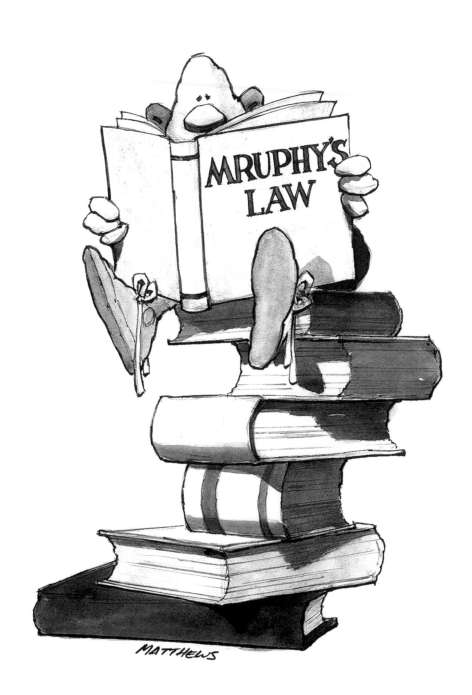

Lessons

Pain

Patterns

Self Talk

Your Mind is a Magnet

Why Set Goals?

Wishing for things

Commitment

A Track Record

Enjoying Your Work

Making More Money

The Law of the Seed

Why Think Positive?

Peace of Mind

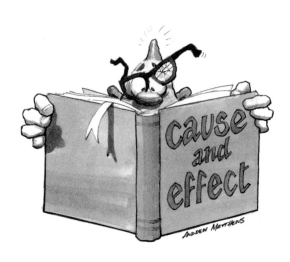

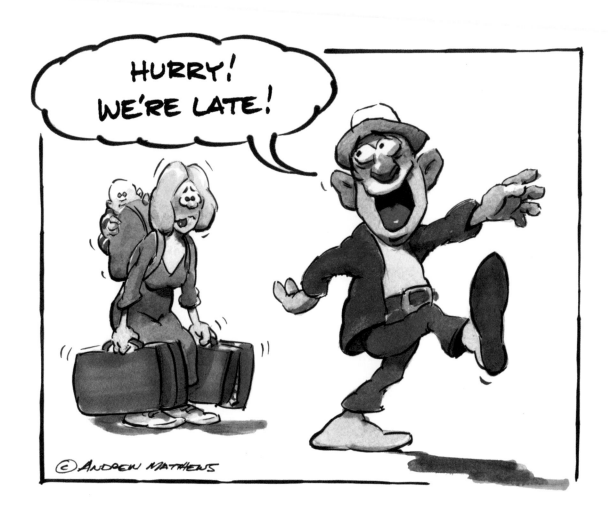

Lessons

Annie is an intelligent, hard-working, attractive lady with a great sense of humour. In the last twenty years she has had a string of relationships with drug addicts who spend her money and drunks who beat her up.

In life, history tends to repeat itself. Until we learn a lesson, we keep getting it again – and again!

IF PEOPLE TAKE ADVANTAGE OF YOU ...
If your friends expect you to solve their problems, carry their stuff, clean their mess, buy their lunch – and you keep doing it – it will keep happening.

IF YOU KEEP GETTING RIPPED OFF ...
If you allow yourself to be cheated by landlords, auto mechanics and repairmen, it will keep happening.

Until you find some courage or learn some skills, you will bleed money.

IF YOU KEEP DATING JERKS ...
If you tolerate rude, lazy, selfish boyfriends – figuring any relationship is better than no relationship – you'll meet an endless stream of "partners from hell".

History repeats itself until we make a stand.

You might say, "If I were somewhere else – maybe Hawaii – or if I had different friends – I wouldn't have these problems!" Yes you would!

When we have a weakness, it's like a magnet ... wherever we go we attract the same lessons. It's a law of life.

Miserable people say, "Why does everything happen to me?"
Effective people say, "I'd better learn this lesson or it will keep coming back!"

IN A NUTSHELL
Assume that every problem in your life is a lesson to make you stronger. Then you never feel like a victim.

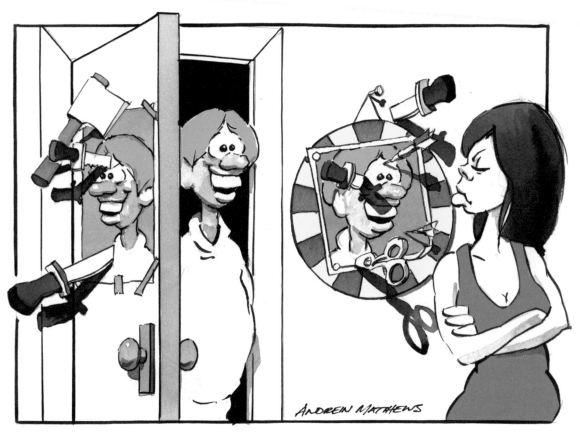

"Did someone make you angry?"

Pain

When you accidentally bite your tongue, it's hard to see "pain" as something positive. The same goes for a blister on your big toe – who needs a throbbing foot?

But what if you felt no pain? How often would you bite off bits of your tongue – or burn your backside in the bath?

Physical pain is a marvellous alarm system that prevents further damage. It tells us: "You'd better change what you're doing!"

Emotional pain gives us a similar message, i.e. "You'd better change how you're thinking!"

It's normal to get angry or jealous or a bit resentful – temporarily. But if those feelings become permanent the message may be:

"Don't expect to control other people."
"Don't expect other people to behave like you."
"Don't depend on other people to make you happy!"

While we keep thinking the same thoughts, we keep feeling the same pain.

(And then we say "But I'm right!" Unfortunately being "right" doesn't help!)

A blister on your foot is a message to change your shoes.

With emotional pain – which feels like a blister on the brain – the message is usually to change your thinking.

IN A NUTSHELL

With both physical and emotional pain, when we keep doing the same thing, it keeps hurting!

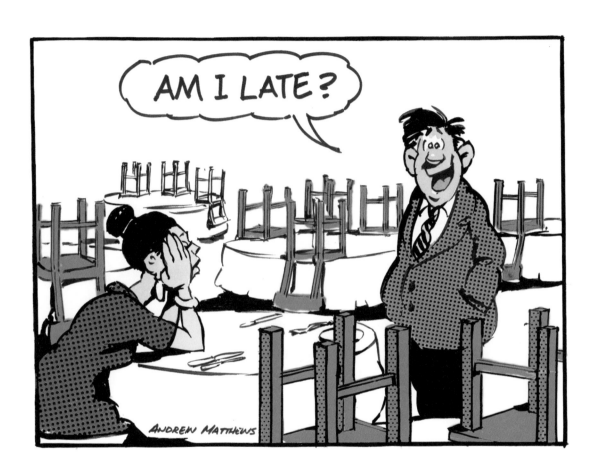

Patterns

Some people are always broke! They win the lottery, and before you know it they need a bank loan to buy a hamburger.

Some people are always late! They can get up at 5.00 am to be at work by 9.00, and at 10.15 they are still searching the house for car keys and brushing their teeth!

Some people make friends wherever they go.
Some people make money wherever they go.
Some people always get sick on vacation.

Why? Because we have subconscious "patterns" of behaviour. Most things we do, we do without thinking – as with breathing or driving a car. We spend all our cash automatically, we make ourselves late automatically.

Now here's the good news ... you are not "your patterns". You can change your subconscious habits with visualisation and mental rehearsal.

Professional sportspeople all use visualisation. Why? Because our brain cells can't tell the difference between a real and an imagined experience. When we visualise perfect behaviour, we program our brain cells for better performance.

It's easy. You simply close your eyes, take some deep breaths and relax, and play mental movies of you performing perfectly. Practise your golf swing in bed. Rehearse your public speaking on the bus – but in your mind!

Regularly picture yourself as organised, confident or performing at your peak. Over weeks and months you'll notice the difference.

It's simple, unsophisticated and it works – for anybody.

IN A NUTSHELL

No one has to stay stuck. If you are serious, you can change old patterns. You're a human being – you're not a tree.

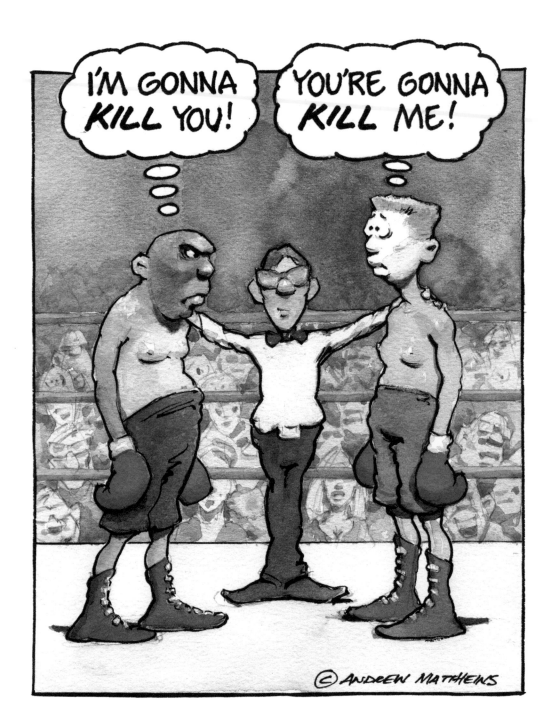

Self-Talk

I knew a guy called Peter. He was forever telling people, "Everything I earn goes to pay bills". He was like a parrot! And no surprise ... he was always broke!

Your language shapes your life. If you tell people you are always broke, you will likely stay broke. If you expect to forget, you will forget! If you expect to behave like an idiot ...

Imagine a boxer stepping into the ring, and telling himself:
"I'm a loser. I'm a chicken!"
How long would he last?
Imagine a singer walking onstage, and telling herself:
"I'm hopeless! They'll hate me!"
How well would she sing?
It's a recipe for disaster.

Yet, lots of us use this same recipe every day. We tell ourselves:
"I'm fat." "I have a lousy memory." "I'm always broke." "I'm an idiot." Then we wonder why we fail!

So how do you start to think positively? The first step is to watch your mouth! Notice what you SAY about yourself.

From today, NEVER SAY ANYTHING BAD ABOUT YOURSELF.
Never tell people: "I'm useless, I always screw up, my boyfriends always dump me ..."

Make a commitment: "From today, I will not criticise myself. If I have nothing good to say about me, I will keep my mouth shut."

It's sometimes hard to control our thoughts – but we CAN control what comes out of our mouth. Once we take control of our language, we begin to have more positive thoughts and life gets better.

IN A NUTSHELL
We become what we think about!

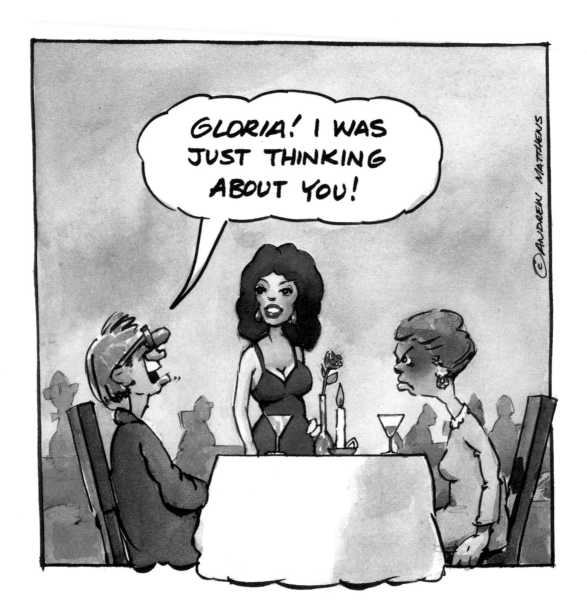

Your Mind is a Magnet

How often do you ...
- bump into old friends in unlikely places?
- learn a new word, and suddenly you see it everywhere?
- hum an old tune, and then hear it on the radio?

How often do you think about someone –
and seconds later they phone you?

Coincidence? Not really.
Your mind is a magnet.

Happy people attract other happy people.
Positive thinkers attract opportunities.
Crooks attract crooks.

Thoughts might be invisible but they are REAL THINGS – just like electricity or gravity. And thought energy obeys natural laws.

If radio waves and TV signals can travel huge distances – through bricks and concrete – why not thoughts? Your brain is at least as amazing as any TV transmitter.

A thousand books have been written on the power of thought. How many "coincidences" do we need to get the message?

If you sweat enough about going broke, it will happen.
If you worry enough about getting sick, it will happen.

Picture yourself surrounded by true friends – and you'll find them.
Picture success, and work toward it, and you are on your way.

IN A NUTSHELL
You attract what you think about.

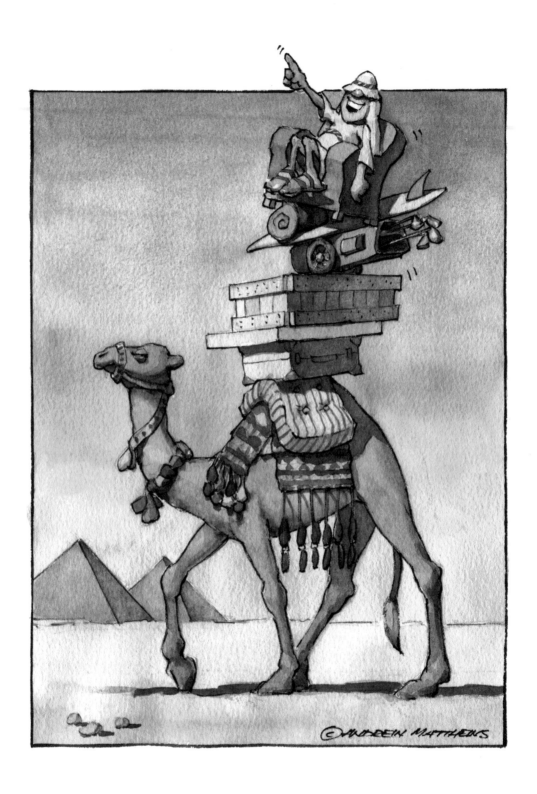

Why Set Goals?

Sometimes we pick up the newspaper and read where a mother of three has just rowed across the Atlantic in a bathtub – or we read about an accountant who is riding a camel from Calcutta to Casablanca.

We might ask ourselves, "Why not take a plane?"

The answer to that is ... If you travel by bathtub (or camel), you arrive a very different person to the one who left!

Not only do you reach your destination knowing a lot more about stars and rain and navigation – you know a lot more about yourself, and about your own courage and capabilities.

Buying a plane ticket doesn't have the same effect.

When you set yourself a goal to run a business or a marathon, when you set a goal to get a degree or a promotion, or to learn Chinese, you arrive a different person to the one who started.

That's what "goals" are really about – what they make of us in the process of achieving them.
That's why we bother.

Your neighbours and your brother-in-law might not understand this concept.

So they ask you, "Why try so hard?"
"Why aim so high?"

The answer is, "For what we become in the process".

IN A NUTSHELL
We set goals not for what we GET, but for what we BECOME.

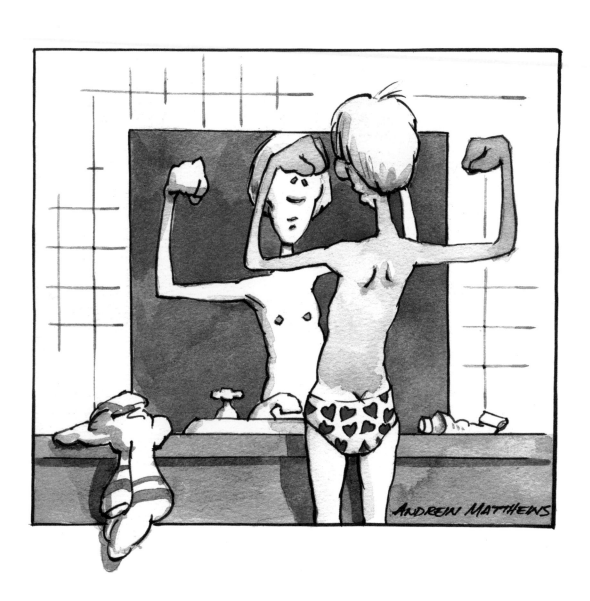

Wishing for Things

Lots of us use visualisation to achieve goals. It's where you:
a) choose a goal, and then
b) continue to imagine yourself with the goal already achieved –
   until you actually achieve it.

Whether you want to lose weight, gain confidence or get better at anything, experts agree that visualisation works. "As you think, so you become." Regularly picturing success – AND putting in the necessary effort – hastens results.

So we might ask, "Why not just WISH for things?" Isn't that similar? No!

Visualising means:
- You choose a goal, eg. a flat stomach, an interesting job, a change of lifestyle.
- You picture your goal already achieved in the present moment.
- This image becomes fixed in your subconscious.
- You continue to work toward your goal.
- You keep moving forwards.

Wishing means:
- You tell yourself, "I hate what I've got."
- You wish for more money, or more happiness or Brad Pitt.
- Your mind drifts around in the future.
- You have no strategy.
- Nothing happens.

KEY POINT: We can only change our life by putting energy into the PRESENT MOMENT. When we wish for things, our mind is in the FUTURE. So the more we wish for things, the more we stay STUCK!

Don't wish! No matter how bad your situation! Set your goal, make a plan, picture your improvement, put in the effort. In the meantime, be happy with what you have got. While you are saving for the Ferrari, be happy with the old clunker.

IN A NUTSHELL

As you think, so you become.
As you wish, so you become ... frustrated.

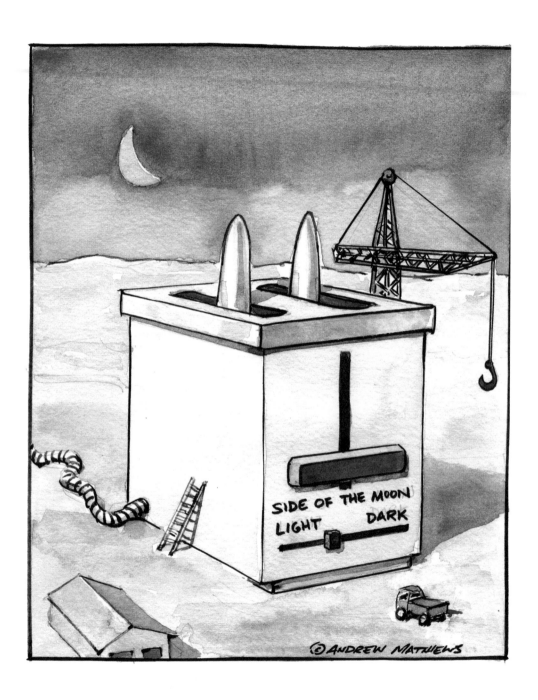

Commitment

When, in 1961, President John F. Kennedy committed to put a man on the moon "before this decade is out", he had no idea how it would be done – and NASA didn't know how either.

A million technical problems had to be solved:

What kind of rockets, engines, landing craft, space suits, underwear do you take to the moon?

Do all the astronauts go straight to the moon or do you leave a guy in a command capsule in lunar orbit?

And if you get to the moon, how do you make sure you don't land in a hole?

How do you get home?

And where do you find two billion dollars to pay for the trip?

The Americans solved each problem, one by one, and in July 1969 the world watched Neil Armstrong take that first giant step.

The Apollo project was like any successful project. Your commitment is the glue that holds it together. First you commit, heart and soul. Then you solve the problems, one at a time.

If you want to build a business, you first commit to it, and then you figure out how to get the customers.

If you want to write a book or get a degree, you commit to it, and then you figure out how to finish it.

The same goes for a marriage – you commit to it, and then day by day, you figure out how to make it work.

You start without all the answers and without any guarantees.

IN A NUTSHELL

To achieve any worthwhile goal, you first decide, "I will do this, whatever it takes".

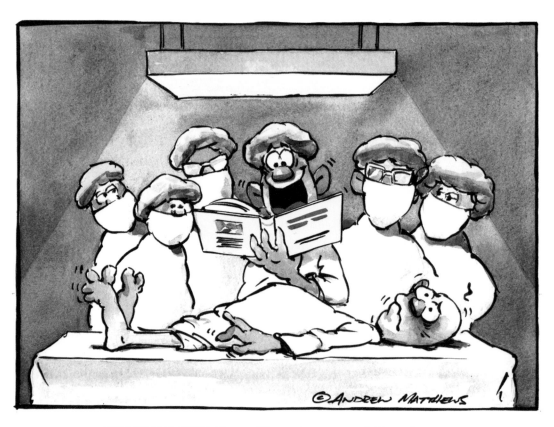

"BRAIN SURGERY: You will need a saw, a drill and some wire or tape. STEP 1: Remove top of head ... see attached illustration of coconut ... "

A Track Record

I know a fellow who is forever trying to clinch million dollar deals. But his big deals never happen! Meanwhile his car is falling apart and even his dog is getting thin.

Why? He never learned to clinch hundred dollar deals!
He never developed the habit of succeeding.

You first learn to catch little fish, then big fish. Surgeons practise on tonsils before they do brain surgery!

Many tycoons start washing cars or selling newspapers at about ten years of age.

Ingvar Kamprad, founder of Ikea, started business as a young boy, selling matches to neighbours from his bicycle. He expanded into fish, Christmas tree decorations and pencils before eventually creating his fold-up furniture empire. Today he is one of the world's richest men.

At age twelve Steven Spielberg started making amateur movies of family camping trips. To finance his films, he charged friends admission while his sister Annie sold popcorn.

You develop a "success pattern", you sharpen your skills and then you aim higher. What's so important about a success pattern?
It's what gets you to BELIEVE IN YOURSELF.
When you know in your heart that:
1. "I've prepared myself for this,"
2. "I can do it!" and
3. "I deserve it", you are on your way.

When you don't believe in yourself, you are dead in the water.

Also, other people's patterns will tell you more about their future than all of their promises and all of their good intentions.

If some guy wants to: a) work for you b) borrow money c) be your business partner or d) give you brain surgery, check his track record.

If there's no success pattern, look out!

IN A NUTSHELL
Wherever you are headed, start small and make success a habit.

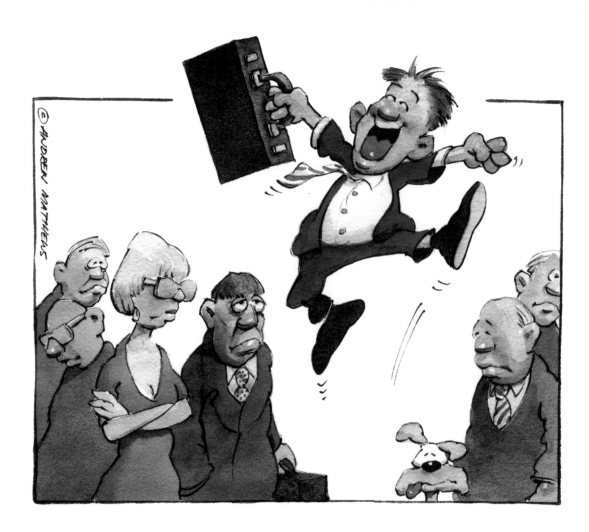

Enjoying Your Work

Recently I saw a TV show about a fellow called P.C. Taylor.

P.C. removes garbage. He and his team clean the subway tunnels in New York City – not the platforms, the underground tubes!

He spends his life in the dirty, stinking, rat-infested, trash-ridden tunnels through which the trains run.

In the documentary they took the cameras underground. It's like being in a long cave, but not so healthy. P.C. has been at this job for 25 years – killing rats and hauling out rubbish.

The interviewer asked P.C., "So do you like your job?"

"Like it?" he said. "I love it!"

He said, "Homeless people live down there in those tunnels. And I'm helping to give them a better home. And while I'm helping the homeless, I'm putting my two daughters through college!"

P.C. is proud of his work. He also proves that it is possible to find job satisfaction in a miserable workplace.

I suspect it's not actually the garbage and the rats that excite him – it is his belief that he is helping to make the world a better place. In other words, it's easier to do a lousy job if you are focused on WHY you do it.

I think of P.C. quite a lot! Whenever I have a job to do that I don't want to do, I imagine myself chasing rats and hauling garbage.

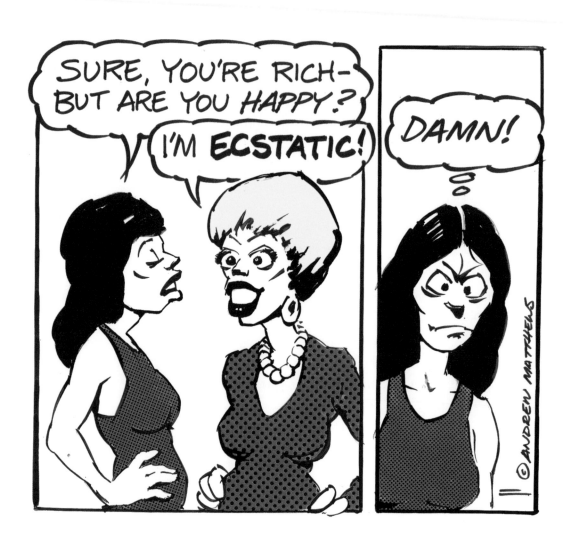

Making More Money

Question: Which people make the most money?

Answer: It's mostly the people who use their imagination to create things ... people like Stephen King who create stories, people like Celine Dion who create music, people like the Ted Turners and Richard Bransons who build organizations and the Oprah Winfreys who create entertainment.

So you say, "If I'm not a creative genius, and I want to make more money, where will it come from?"
Answer: "From your imagination – whoever you are."

Example: Let's say that you are broke and living on bread and water. You ask yourself, "How can I eat some healthy food and save money?"
Strategy: "I'll grow bean sprouts in my kitchen for virtually nothing!"

After a month of eating sprouts you figure, "I hate sprouts! I'll sell my sprouts to the neighbours for a dollar a bag, and buy steak!" Ideas solve your money problems!

Example: You are already working for a boss but you want to make money in your spare time.
Strategy: You ask yourself, "What skills have I got – or what do I love to do – that people will pay me to do?" You imagine yourself making personalised greeting cards or walking the neighbours' dogs. You imagine yourself renovating your apartment or teaching aerobics.

You try some ideas. Eventually one works. Where did it all begin? In your imagination.

If you already have your own business, increased profits will likely depend on how imaginatively you answer questions like ... "How can I do more with less?" "How can I manage my time better?"
"What do people really want – and how can I deliver it?"

And guess what! Many of your ideas won't work. Fortunately, you don't need every idea to work – just one or two.

IN A NUTSHELL
If money comes from your imagination, it is not necessarily working harder that will make you more money – it is an increase in the quantity and the quality of your ideas.

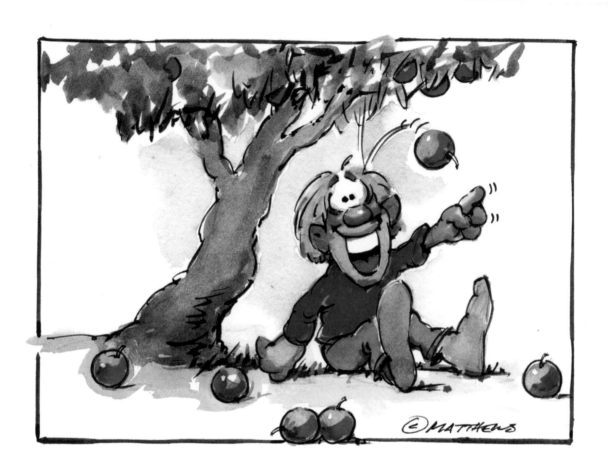

The Law of the Seed

The first book book I ever wrote was a children's book. I had heard that getting a book published can be tough, so I got the addresses of sixty children's publishers, made sixty copies of my manuscript and sent them all over the world.

I felt really smart! I thought, "Worst case scenario I'll get fifty rejections and then choose from the rest".

Guess how many rejections I got! Sixty-one!! One publisher wrote to me twice!

So I wrote another book and sent that one out to publishers. Eventually someone said, "Yes!"

If we really want to make something happen, we usually need to try more than once.

It is a principle of nature.

Let's say an apple tree bears five hundred apples, each with ten seeds. We might say, "That's a lot of seeds! Why would you need so many seeds to grow just a few more trees?

Because most seeds never grow.

In your life this principle might mean:
You'll need to attend twenty interviews to get one job.
You'll interview forty people to find one good employee.
You'll talk to fifty people to sell one house, car, vacuum cleaner, insurance policy, idea.

And you might need to meet a hundred acquaintances to find one special friend.

When we understand the "Law of the Seed", we stop feeling like victims. We don't get so disappointed.

The laws of nature are not things to take personally. We just need to understand them – and work with them.

IN A NUTSHELL
Successful people fail more often. They plant more seeds.

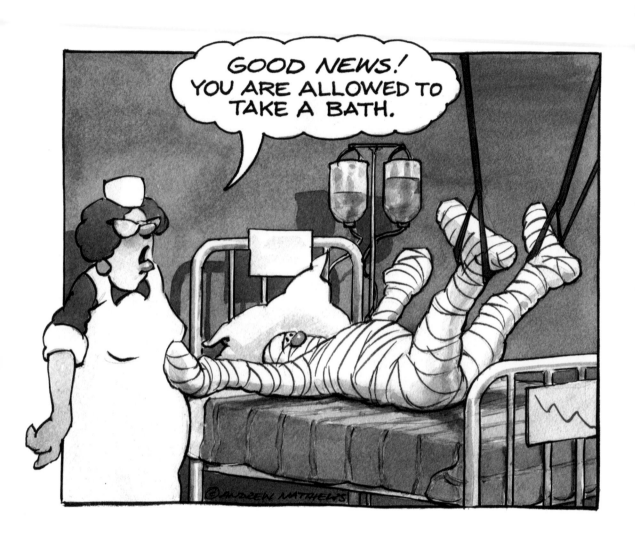

Why Think Positive?

When things go wrong, remember:

It's not WHAT HAPPENS TO YOU that matters most.
It's how YOU THINK ABOUT what happens to you ...

EXAMPLE:

Let's say that you are at the airport, waiting to catch a flight, and the airline tells you, "Sorry! Mechanical trouble. You won't be leaving for three hours!"

You are furious. You tell yourself:
"This is terrible! This is a disaster!"

While you remain stressed, things will get worse!
People will trip over you, spill coffee in your lap and lose your baggage.
When you fight life, life always wins!

Then finally you cool down. You tell yourself:
"There's nothing I can do about it. I'll make the most of it."

Suddenly, everything changes! From nowhere an old friend appears, or you make a new friend, or you stumble on a fresh opportunity –
and life begins to support you.

Once we change our thoughts about "a bad situation", we can take advantage of it.
Life's great opportunities mostly arrive disguised as misfortune and disaster.

EXAMPLE:

Imagine two women, Mary and Jane. Both get divorced.
Mary says, "I've failed. My life is over."
Jane says, "My life has just begun!"
Who will blossom?

IN A NUTSHELL

Every "disaster" in your life is not so much a disaster, as a situation waiting for you to change your mind about it.

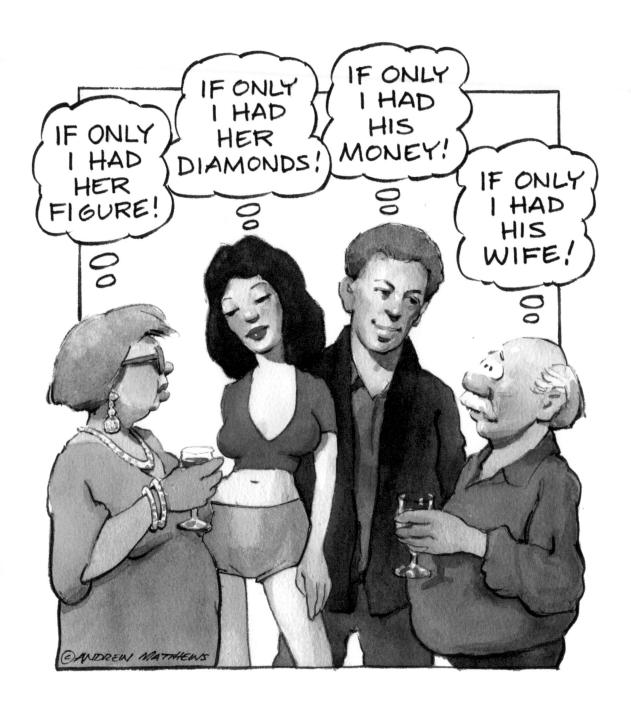

Peace of Mind

If you ask your neighbour,
"What would give you peace of mind?" he might tell you,
"A vacation in Bermuda!" or
"An extra hundred grand would give me peace!", or
"A new Ferrari would make me content!"

But going places – and getting stuff – is usually a temporary
solution ...

Let's say you buy a lottery ticket and by some miracle you win your
dream Ferrari. Today you are content. Tomorrow you are saying, "If I could just
catch that little punk who scratched it in the car park!"

Peace of mind rarely comes from getting more stuff.
Getting more stuff usually leads to wanting even more stuff!

Peace of mind starts with being grateful for what you have right now.

GRATITUDE is POWER, and here's why ...

When you are thankful for what you have – for the friends you have, and for the
things you've got – you attract more good people and good things.

People who always complain about what they DON'T HAVE,
stay stuck.
Complainers attract more things to complain about!

It is a law of life. It's hard to explain, but you can observe it around you. We get
more of what we dwell upon.

That's why all the spiritual masters have taught the same lesson ...
"Start by being thankful. Be happy with what you have now,
and more will come to you." It's practical advice.

IN A NUTSHELL

Every time you say a silent "thank you" you become
more peaceful – and more powerful.

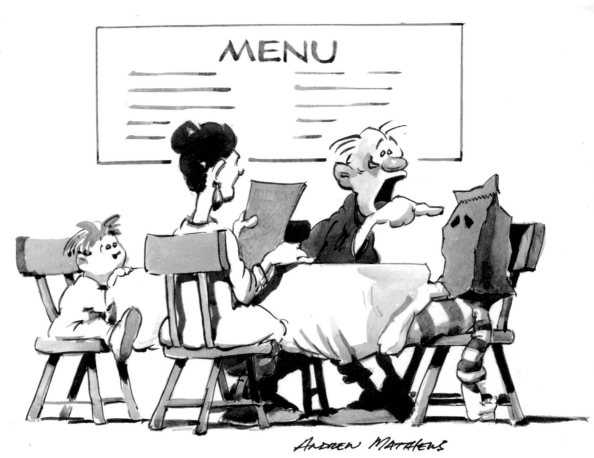

"When I was a teenager, I was **proud** to be seen with my parents!"

Relationships

Family

Compliments

Trying to Change People

Forgiving People

Friends and Money

Presents

Other People's Relationships

"Make Me Happy!"

"I Love You!"

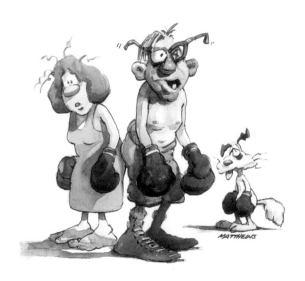

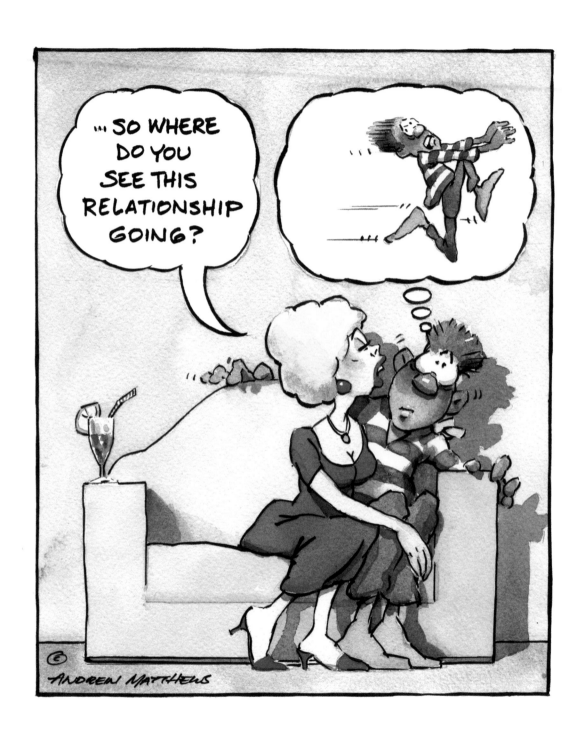

Relationships

Relationships are tricky!

The strategies we think SHOULD work, don't work!
The strategies we think WON'T work, do work ...

Impressing people:
When we try to impress people - by proving that we are clever or rich or cool - people can see through us. And then we look silly.

We usually impress other people when we AREN'T TRYING to. That's why babies and animals and very old people are so appealing. They don't care what you think - they are perfectly natural.

Chasing people:
When we chase girlfriends, boyfriends - even dogs - they run away! Why? Because we are chasing them!

When we try to trap people in relationships, they can't wait to escape!
When we LET GO of people, they often come back!

Helping people:
When we try to help others - children, friends, employees – by solving their problems, they become dependent on us – and even lazy! The more we help, the less they do.

Mostly, we help people by NOT HELPING too much.

Getting people's attention:
When we are desperate to be heard, we shout at people. And the louder we shout, the less they hear. Strangely, the opposite works.

People pay attention to us when we LISTEN.

IN A NUTSHELL
There's such a thing as trying too hard!

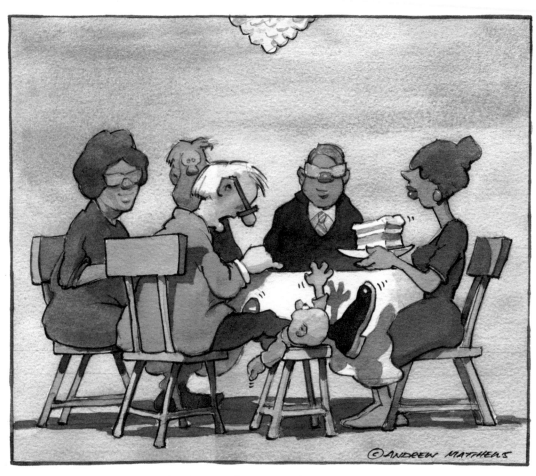

"Steven's had enough to eat - haven't you Steven?"

Family

Isn't it funny how we tend to treat strangers a whole lot better than we treat family?

We want our friends to think well of us. We listen more attentively to casual acquaintances – and we have more time for them – than we do for our children or our parents!

Parents make daily sacrifices for us and we hardly give it a second thought.

On the other hand, small favours from strangers become etched in our memory!

Have you ever invited complete strangers to dinner? Here's what happens ...

You spend four hours shopping and you blow the entire week's grocery budget. You take a whole afternoon to set the table with your best silver and crockery. You borrow fancy glassware from the neighbours.

You dig out the candles. You wash the dog.

You serve a spectacular seafood banquet ... and you never see those people again!

Next week, Mum and Dad come over and they get leftovers ... a chicken in a paper bag!

Perhaps we should turn it around sometimes. Save the lobster and champagne for Mum and Dad – and when strangers come to dinner, say, "Sorry about the chicken in the bag. You should have been here last week. Mum and Dad came over!"

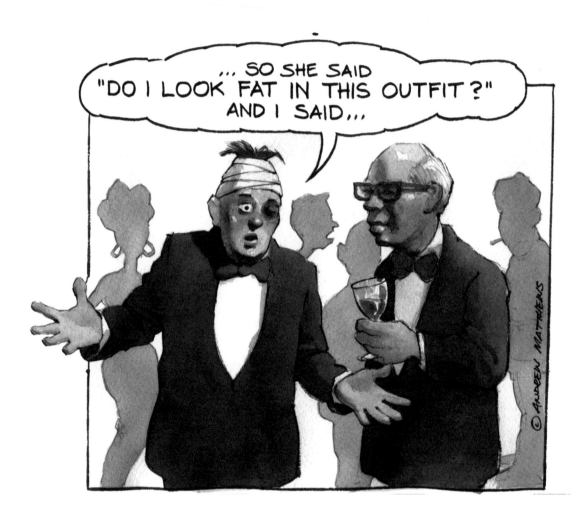

Compliments

My wife, Julie went to the local seafood shop last month. A young fellow called David took the order. David was polite, helpful and took great care in preparing for us a beautiful side of salmon.

Next day Julie wrote a letter to David thanking him for his professional service - and she also sent a copy to his boss. David was over the moon and his boss was also delighted. How many thank-you letters do you think fish sellers get? David has since been promoted.

Most people feel that their efforts go unnoticed. Most people feel under-loved. So when you give them a compliment like:
"You do great work!"
"That is a stunning outfit!"
"You are an inspiring teacher."
"You have a beautiful smile!"
you light up their day – or their whole month!

Of course, some people are embarrassed by compliments.
They might even disagree with you.
But you can bet they appreciate your kind words –
they just don't know how to say, "thank you".
Compliment them anyway!

And here's the big bonus to giving compliments:
It makes YOU happier.

One key point on giving praise ... a compliment is different from flattery! Flattery is insincere. A compliment is SINCERE RECOGNITION of someone's qualities. People know the difference.

Want to be happier?
Every day, aim to give one person a compliment.

In life, you find what you look for.
If you look for good things, you find them.
If you look for faults, you find them.

IN A NUTSHELL
Your happiness depends on what you DECIDE to notice.

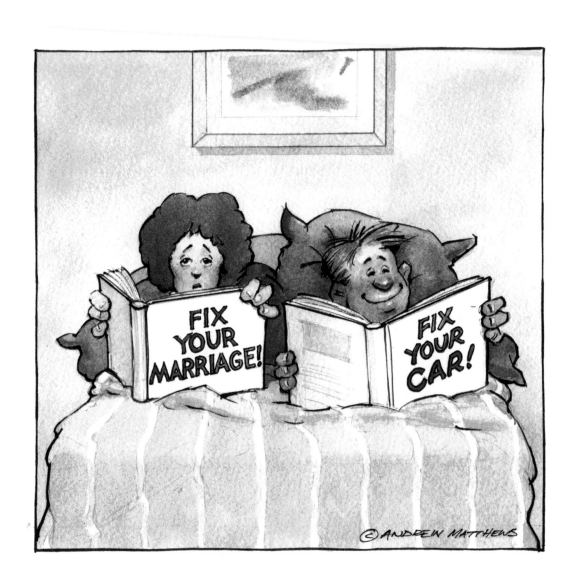

Trying to Change People

Trying to change people is mostly a bad idea! Why?
Because it doesn't work. You get frustrated and they hate you!

Example 1:

Take Mary and Fred. They are lovers.
Mary figures, "Fred's not perfect but I can CHANGE him! I'll teach him manners, I'll stop him drinking ..."
Mary is determined to "fix" Fred. But Fred doesn't want to be fixed.
So Fred gets angry and resentful – and Mary gets exhausted.

Example 2:

Let's say that my life is a mess.
I'm out of control, and everyone can see it.
Friends give me advice, and I ignore it.
Soon enough ... KABOOM!
I get fired, I go bankrupt ... or I get arrested.
I am shattered! But BECAUSE I am shattered, I start to pay attention!
I change my behaviour. I change my life!

Positive change is a natural process. Frequently it unfolds like this:
Step 1: stupidity, followed by
Step 2: disaster
Step 3: desperation, and finally
Step 4: wisdom.

We need each step. If you force change upon others, you disrupt the process.
You say, "But it's painful to watch other people being STUPID!"
Right! But if you force them to change, they don't learn.

(Parents and policemen sometimes need to force people!
Most other times, we best let others make their own mistakes.)

IN A NUTSHELL

People fall into two groups:
a) Those who make regular adjustments to their life strategy
b) Those who like to hit a brick wall, and then change.

Neither want you to tell them how to live!

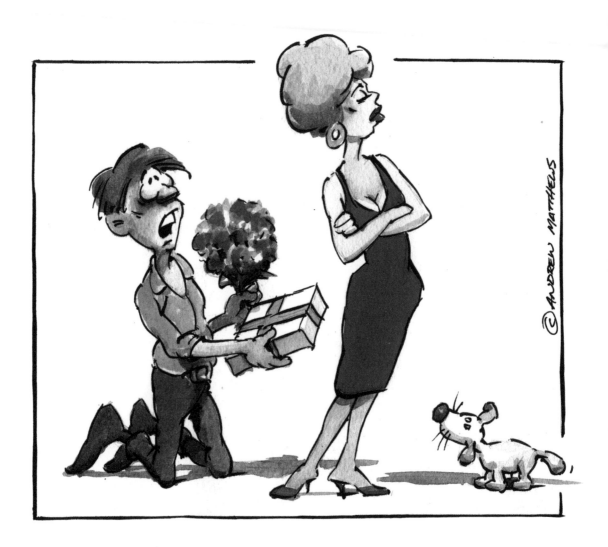

Forgiving People

Growing up, I remember hearing my Mum, and various "religious" people, telling me that it is a good idea to forgive people – that forgiveness is 'holy' or 'spiritual'.

But there is a more basic reason to forgive people: when you don't forgive them, it ruins your life!

Let's say:
    a)   you are my boss and you give me the sack, or
    b)   you are my girl, and you run off with my buddy.
So I say, "I'll never forgive you for that!"

Who suffers? Not you!

I'm pacing the floor. I've got the knot in my stomach. I'm losing sleep.

You are probably out partying!

Where do we get the idea that if WE don't forgive people, THEY suffer? It's nuts!

Recent studies at the Public Health Institute in California confirm that hostility and resentment tear down your immune system and double your risk of heart attack, cancer and even diabetes. Bitterness makes you sick!

To forgive someone, you don't have to agree with what they did.

You just have to want your own life to work.

IN A NUTSHELL

Is forgiveness easy? Usually not.
But you don't forgive people for their benefit.
You do it for your benefit.

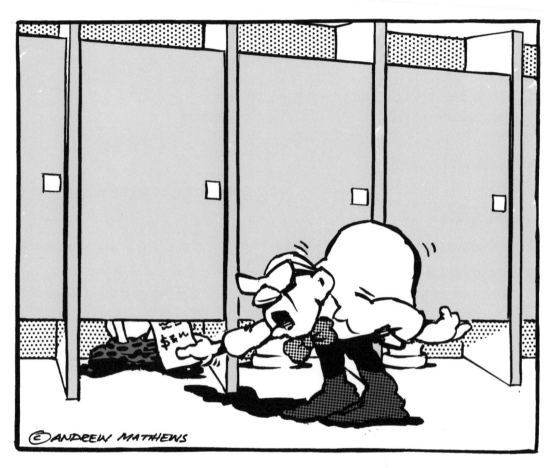

" Sir, your friends at table 6 say it's your turn to buy lunch. "

Friends and Money

I know a guy called Jim. Jim has worked hard all his life and he is worth millions.

Jim lives the good life. He travels a lot, enjoys good food and wine, and loves entertaining his friends. Jim is easy going and generous.

Recently, Jim told me about one of his friends, Ted, who is usually broke. He said, "I like Ted. Ted often stays in our home and we also take him on vacation. I have treated him to a hundred meals in some wonderful restaurants. You know what bugs me? Not once in ten years has he bought me a meal or a hamburger, or a lousy coffee!"

Guess what! Even wealthy people keep count!
Even generous people count!

It's not necessarily the dollars they worry about. It's the attitude. It's being taken for granted.

Ted figures, "Jim is rich. Someone has to pay. It may as well be him!"

So far, Jim hasn't complained. But he's had enough. And any day now, Ted is going to lose a friend – and Ted will ask himself, "What happened?"

Amongst your friends, you know who are the first to reach for their wallets, who are last to reach for their wallets – and who always forget their wallets.

You also know who'll be in the bathroom when the bill arrives!

And do you know what? Your friends have you figured out too!

IN A NUTSHELL

If your friends are richer than you, and all you have to spend on them is a dollar, spend that dollar!

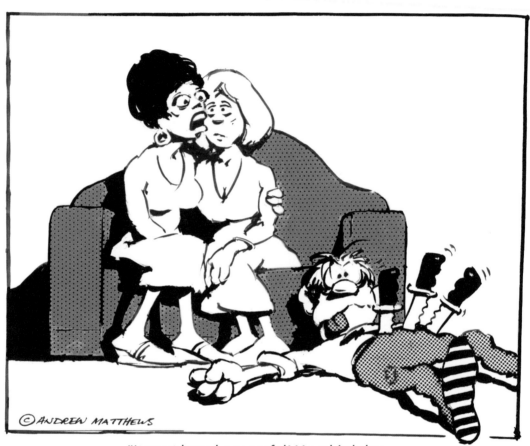

"It must have been awful! Your birthday ...
and he gives you stupid steak knives!"

Presents

Tony's wife wanted him to buy her a new ironing board. It was early February. So he waited a week and gave it to her on Valentines Day. Bad idea!

Guys often get into trouble for buying their wives and girlfriends the wrong presents. So this page is for the guys. It is based on my serious dinner party research ...

Guys, when you receive a birthday present, like a hammer drill, you say to yourself, "Great – this is really practical. I can use this!" So when you go shopping for your wife's birthday present, you look for something "useful". Big mistake!

Rule #1.

In general: Guys like presents that are USEFUL. Women like presents that are PERSONAL. Though some women like to get vacuum cleaners and can openers for their birthdays, most hate useful presents!

We guys should have gotten the message by now! In those romantic movies, when the couple kiss on the beach, and he says "I'll love you forever and ever", he usually pulls out earrings, roses, pearls, diamonds ... he doesn't give her an electric frypan!

To women, useful presents mean, "You don't REALLY love me!" Other items that aren't personal include coffee grinders and accounting software!

Rule #2

TIMING IS CRITICAL!

With men, it doesn't matter WHEN you get the present. If a guy wants spanners, any time is a good time ... on his birthday, between birthdays, at anniversaries. Give a guy an angle grinder as a get well present and he'll love it! With women, timing usually matters.

Most women feel that they do more than their share of pampering to the men in their lives. They see birthdays and anniversaries as opportunities for us men to show some extra consideration in return.

IN A NUTSHELL

Women want to feel that you were thinking of them – and that you made a special effort. It's usually not about cost.

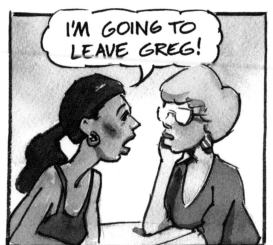

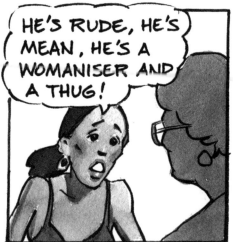

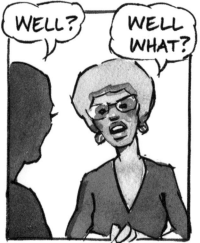

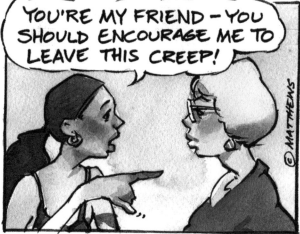

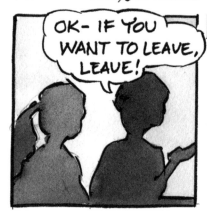

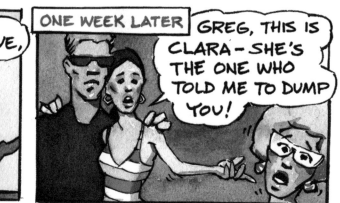

Other People's Relationships

Has this ever happened to you ...

Two friends of yours decide to split up.
They ask for your advice.
You tell them what you think. You try to help.

Next week they are back together again – and they both hate you!

What's the lesson here?

Be careful when offering friends advice on their relationships!

It's a minefield!

IN A NUTSHELL

The only people who REALLY know what is going on in a relationship are the two people in it!

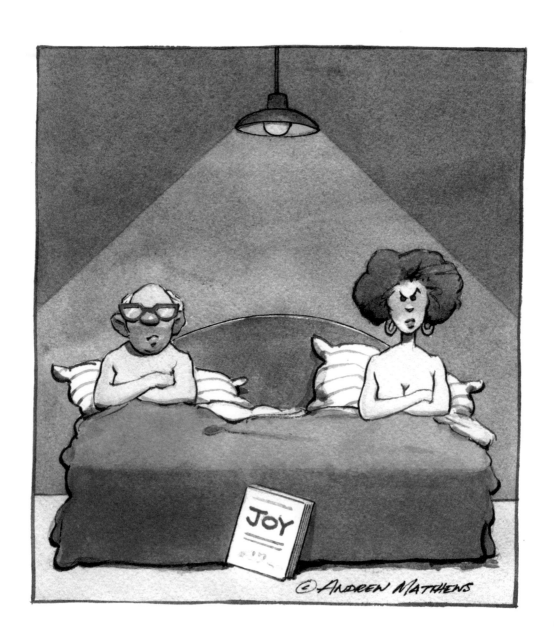

"Make Me Happy!"

When you are feeling cheerful, do you ever say to yourself, "I should go hang out with some gloomy people!"?

You don't! You look for other happy people.
Happy people attract happy people.

Miserable people attract miserable people.

And no one else can ever MAKE you happy!

Where do we get the idea that someone else can MAKE us happy? Maybe from songs and movies ...

In songs and movies people say, "Before you, I was lonely, I was a loser – but you changed everything!"

In the real world people say, "Before you, I was miserable - but you made it WORSE!"

In the real world, other people don't change our lives.
We do it ourselves.

If you are feeling down or depressed, only you can change your thoughts. Step by step, you pull yourself out of the hole.

As you begin to look on the bright side, you attract happy friends and colleagues.

To be surrounded by positive people, you first put a smile on your own face.

IN A NUTSHELL

Your mission in life is not to change the world – just to change yourself.

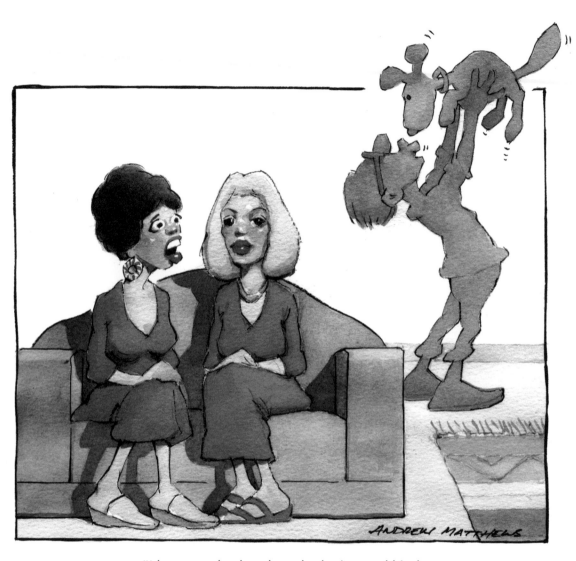

"I know my husband can be loving and kind -
he's that way with the dog!"

"I Love You"

*"Little things I should have said and done
I just never took the time
You were always on my mind ..."*

What is the theme of almost every song and novel, and every movie ever made? LOVE! Lost love, found love, puppy love, risky love, scorned love ...

Nearly everything we do is an attempt to get more love. We buy cool clothes, flash cars and climb the corporate ladder. We do crash diets, get botox, and pierce our body parts.

We figure, "If I look sexy, people will love me."
"If I am clever, people will love me."
"If I am 97% wrinkle free, people will love me."

Every person you'll ever meet is aching for love and acceptance - and some of us are doing crazy things to get it. We get so busy trying to find love that we sometimes forget to tell the people we care about how we feel ...

Fred says, "I told my wife last month that I love her. Can't she remember?" She remembers, Fred, but she wants to be told every month. Actually, wants to be told every day!

Little Johnny is born. For the first few years, Dad gives him endless hugs and tells him, "Daddy loves you!"

Then, when Johnny is about twelve, Dad decides, "He's a big boy now". Dad's cuddles evaporate and Johnny is left wondering, "What did I do wrong? Doesn't he love me any more?"

I've lost count of the number of grown men who have said to me at one time or another: "All I wanted my whole life was for my Dad to tell me that he loved me."

Too often we wait for a tragedy before we tell people what they always wanted to hear. Sometimes the tragedy means it's too late to tell them.

IN A NUTSHELL

To say "I love you" costs so little. And when it is too difficult to say, "I love you", "thank you" is a good start.

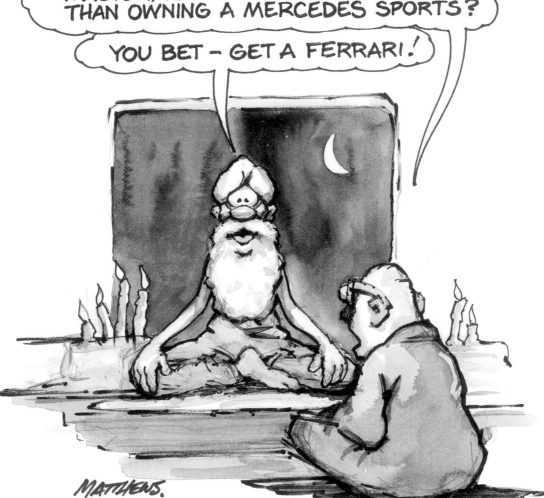

What Is Most Important?

What Surrounds You

Excuses

"I Can't Do It!"

Get Serious

Focus on What You Want

Just Ask

Throw out the Junk!

Prosperity

Save First!

Just do it!

Your Best

When to Quit?

What We Have

Everything Is Connected!

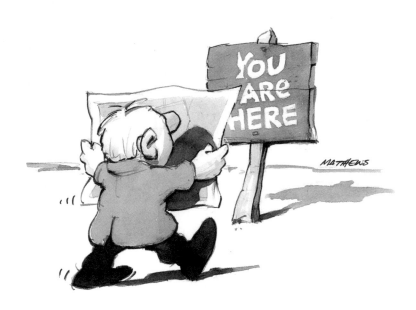

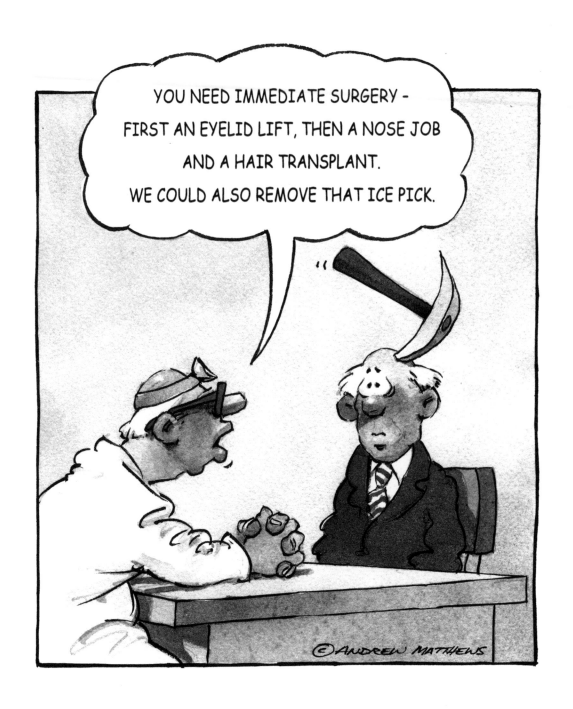

What Is Most Important?

20% of the food you eat creates 80% of the fat!
20% of your neighbours make 80% of the noise.
20% of the people in your office do 80% of the work.
This is the 80/20 rule. You'll see it everywhere!

In 1897 an Italian economist called Pareto discovered that 20% of people in England had 80% of the money. He also found that 20% of pea pods in his garden produced 80% of his peas. Now he is famous!

His Pareto Principle predicts that in any situation, just a few things are much more important than all the rest.

This means:
In business: 20% of customers give you 80% of the profits.
Look after that 20%!

For students: 20% of a book's pages contain 80% of the information.
Concentrate on that 20% - then read the next book.

For you: YOUR DAILY TASKS ARE NOT EQUALLY IMPORTANT. If you have ten jobs to do today, two of them will be more critical than the other eight!

Every day, figure out the 20%. Do those things FIRST.

Simply making a "to do list" is not good enough. Unless you target the 20%, you can waste 80% of your time!

Average people put average effort into lots of things.

Achievers put major effort into key things.

You can't do everything - but you can do the 20%. Don't lose sleep over the 80%.

IN A NUTSHELL

It's not just the amount of effort that matters, but where you put it.

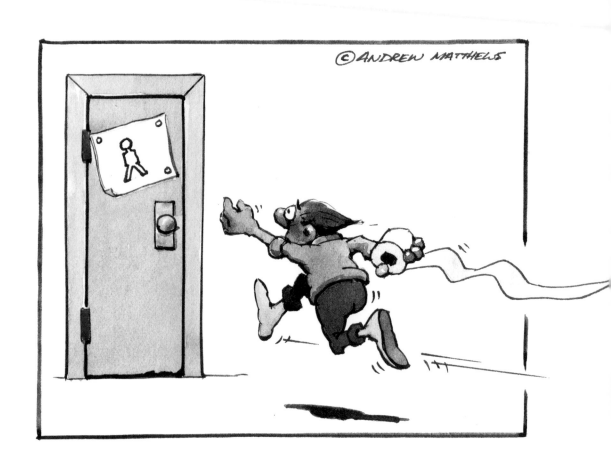

What Surrounds You

Did you ever walk into a public washroom that smelt so bad that you wanted to choke? But you were so desperate to go to the bathroom you had to carry on.

Did you notice something?
By the time you left five minutes later, it didn't smell quite so bad!

And what if you had accidentally locked yourself in there for an hour?
You might be saying, "What smell?"

There's a principle operating here. We get used to our environment!

Live with miserable people, and you become miserable – and you think it's normal!

Work with critical people, and you become critical – and you think it's normal.

If your friends tell lies, it worries you – in the beginning.
Eventually you get used to people telling lies.
Hang out with them long enough and you'll tell some yourself!

Mix with happy and motivated people, and you become happy and motivated - and you think that is normal.

If your family is negative and miserable, then you need to find some bright, happy friends. Somewhere in your life, you need positive company or the pessimists will drag you down – and you won't even know it is happening.

IN A NUTSHELL

We are all affected – and infected – by the people and attitudes around us.

Sometimes we need to take action – or change the company we keep – while we can still notice: "Something smells around here!"

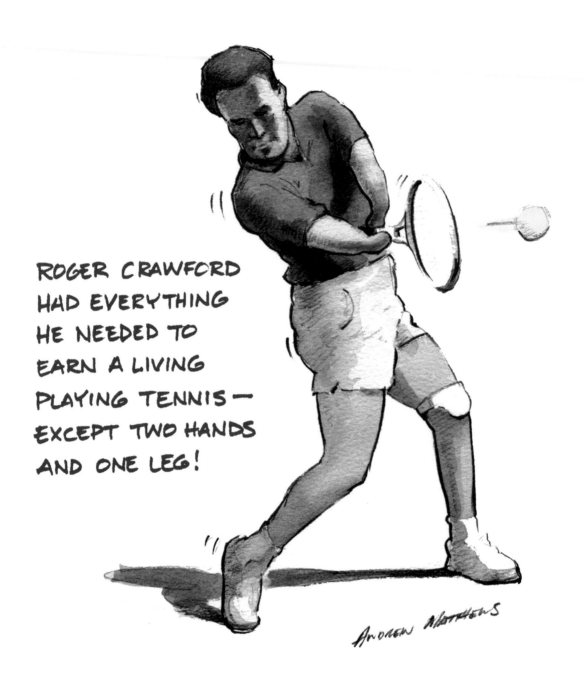

ROGER CRAWFORD
HAD EVERYTHING
HE NEEDED TO
EARN A LIVING
PLAYING TENNIS —
EXCEPT TWO HANDS
AND ONE LEG!

Excuses

In life we have either EXCUSES or we have RESULTS. It seems that some people are here just to teach us that ...

Roger Crawford was born with one leg and two arms, but no hands. What does he do? He's a professional tennis player. That is, he earned professional status and he makes his living playing and coaching tennis.

Digital Dan, of Ferndale, California was a carpenter until he got cancer of the throat and had his voice box removed. When he could no longer speak, he became a disc jockey! Dan types his words into a laptop computer, and the laptop does the talking!

How often do we say, "I'm too old, too tired, too lazy, too busy, it's too hard!"

In 1996 American cyclist Lance Armstrong contracted testicular cancer. When it spread to his abdomen, lungs and brain, doctors gave him a forty percent chance of survival. But Armstrong did more than survive. He got back on his bike and won the world's toughest road race – the Tour de France – six consecutive times, from 1999 to 2004.

Lance has a habit of proving that old saying: "Whatever doesn't kill you makes you stronger."

People like Roger, Dan and Lance remind us that our excuses are mostly cop-outs!

Take any goal you want to achieve ... a university degree, an apartment of your own, a happy marriage, a flat stomach ... and you'll find a hundred reasons why it is inconvenient or impossible.   But all you need is ONE really good reason why you want something! Then you go and get it!

When you want something enough, you find a way. Nothing worthwhile comes without struggle. There's always a story behind the story.

IN A NUTSHELL
Success is not about "the facts". It's about your attitude.

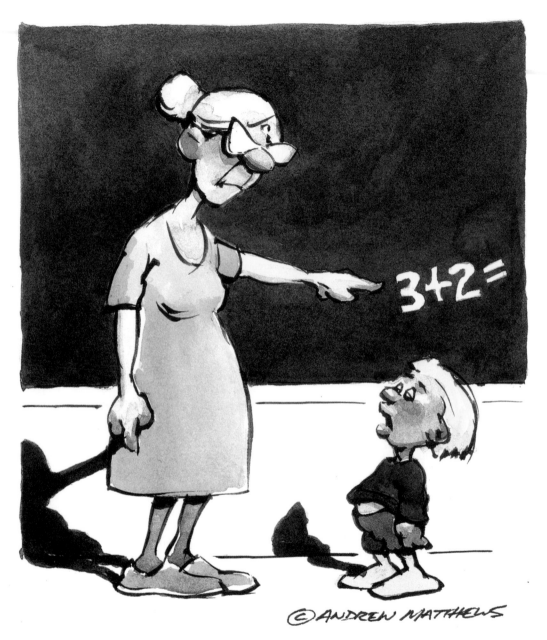

"If I give you the answers, how will you ever learn?"

"I Can't Do It!"

Imagine this story ...

During your first weeks of school, you are sitting in mathematics class gazing out the window when the teacher asks you, "What's the answer?"

"What's the answer?" You don't even know the question! You are speechless. Your face turns red. Panic and tears! At that moment you tell yourself, "I hate mathematics!"

That night your mother asks: "How was school?"
You say: "I couldn't answer the maths question."
And Mother says: "Relax – no one in our family can do mathematics!"

Suddenly you breathe a huge sigh of relief, "Of course I hate multiplication! It's in my genes!"

Soon you are telling your friends, "I hate mathematics. My entire family is bad with numbers!" You figure, "Why make an effort? I'll never conquer it!"

But what REALLY happened here? You got a bad start and fell behind.

Maybe this mathematics story didn't happen to you. But most of us have our own story - about singing, hitting a ball, drawing a picture, about public speaking.

We got a bad start and fell behind. No one came along to encourage us. After one embarrassing experience we gradually convinced ourselves, "I can't do it!"

Do you have fixed ideas about what you CAN and CAN'T DO?
Where did you get these ideas? Are they facts?"

IN A NUTSHELL

When we give ourselves a second chance, and get some help, very often WE CAN DO IT!

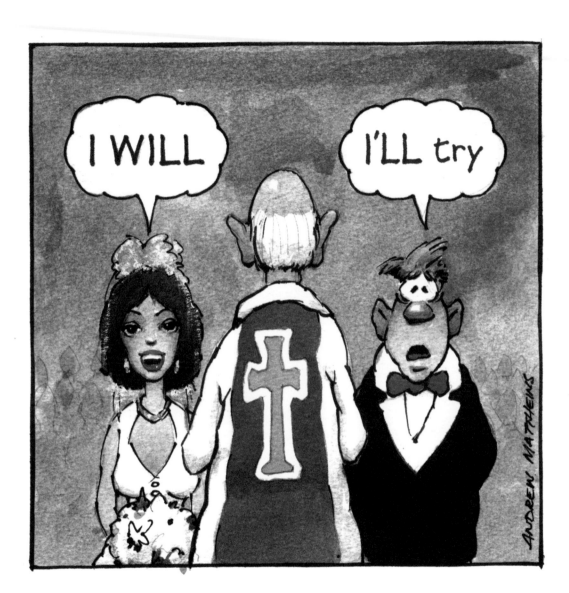

Get SERIOUS!

You will notice something about weak people.
They use weak language!

They use certain words a lot, like "TRY" ...
"I'll TRY to lose weight."
"I'll TRY to get out of debt."

The minute someone says, "I'll TRY", you know that they are only half serious.
When friends say, "I'll TRY to be there", you know they won't show up!

Our words tell people how determined we are.

Parents who tell their children, "TRY to be quiet!", "TRY to behave!" aren't serious. So what do their kids do? Whatever they want!

Instead of telling your children – or your staff –
"You must TRY", say "You must DO IT!"

Instead of telling yourself, "I'LL TRY", tell yourself "I WILL!"
It is challenging – and it will get you much better results ...
"I WILL finish this." "I WILL be happy!"

"I'LL TRY" says, "I'll do this thing if it isn't too hard".
"I WILL" says, "I'll do this thing whatever it takes".

This is not a detail.
It's the difference between casual and committed.
Often, it's the difference between success and failure.

If you want people to believe in you – and if you want to believe in yourself – you have to sound serious!

IN A NUTSHELL
Your words shape your future.

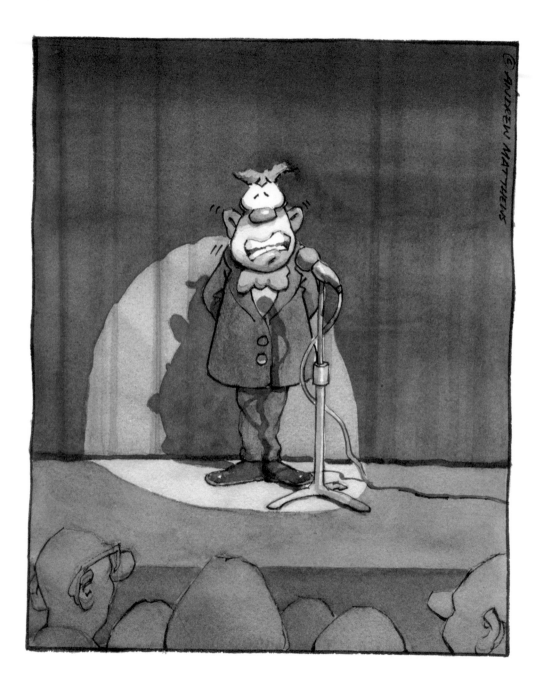

Focus on What You Want

You are about to make a speech in front of two hundred people You tell yourself, "Don't be nervous! Don't forget your lines! Don't embarrass yourself!" Then you get onstage and what happens? You screw it up! You even forget your wife's name!

Why does this happen when you told yourself NOT to be an idiot? It's because of the way our minds work. There is an important principle operating here and it is rarely explained ...

Your mind operates on pictures. To do anything you need a picture. To touch your nose, you need a picture in your mind of your finger on your nose. With this correct picture, your subconscious mind can tell the muscles to do it.

To give a confident speech, you need a picture in your head of you giving a confident speech before you even stand up. Only then can your mind instruct your body to act it out.

You cannot give your mind a message NOT to do something. Your subconscious mind must have a picture of WHAT YOU WANT.

So if you tell yourself, "Don't be nervous!" you automatically fill your subconscious mind with pictures of you shaking and stammering - and that becomes your performance! It's the law of the mind.

What happens when you are on the golf course, at the water hazard, and you tell yourself, "DON'T HIT THE WATER!"? Even though you tell yourself, "Don't hit the water!" your subconscious mind still has only one picture – of your ball taking a swim. And what you see in your mind is what you get.

This explains why confidence is so critical in anything you do. When you are confident, you have only positive pictures in your mind – of a good speech, of a relaxed job interview, of a successful driving test. When you are confident, you don't play disaster movies, you play success movies - so you regularly succeed. You are not perfect, but you always give yourself the best possible chance.

IN A NUTSHELL

Positive thinkers have the habit of picturing what they want, not what they fear! What you think is what you get.

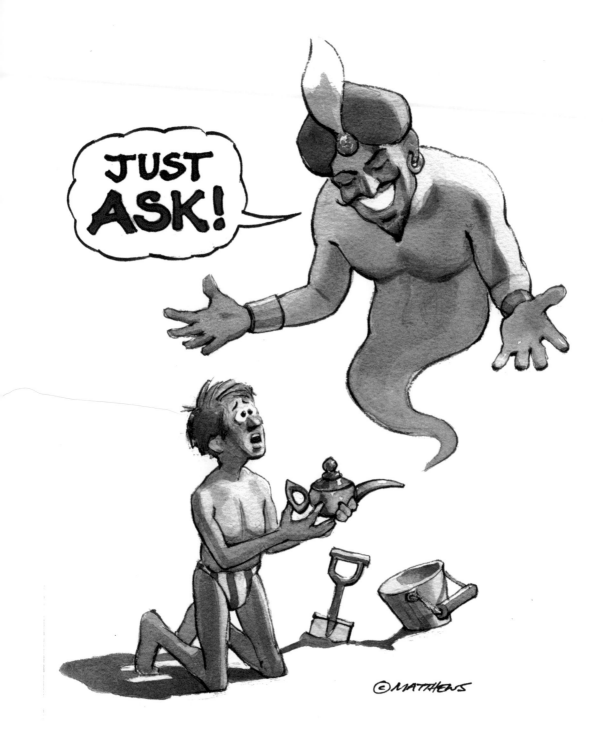

Just Ask!

It was 11am on a Sunday and I was due to catch a plane to Singapore at 2.30pm. Next day in Singapore I was to give a speech to 5,000 people. Suddenly I realised that I had lost my passport.

Julie said, "I'll get you a passport!" She grabbed the phone and started calling emergency immigration numbers all over Australia, but all she got were answering machines or people who said, "Impossible on a Sunday!".

Finally, after 25 calls, Julie spoke to a government official who was at home suffering from a severe hangover. Julie convinced this person to crawl out of bed, drive to the Australian passport office in Currie St., Adelaide, turn off the entire twenty-storey security system, fire up the computers and make a passport for me by 1pm.

Julie is amazing for many reasons. One of them is: she knows how to ask. Julie once rebuilt an orphanage in Indonesia with no money. She visited CEOs of corporations all over Jakarta and asked for donations of bricks, timber, plumbing, paint, roofing iron and labour. Once the orphanage was complete, she kept it supplied with drugs and bandages using the same strategy.

Julie's philosophy is:
1. If you ask, you'll often get.
2. If someone says "No", don't take it personally. Ask someone else.

YOUR success and happiness depend on you asking for things. For small things ... "May I have a refund, an upgrade, can you reschedule my appointment?" "Will you go out with me on a date?"
And for big things ... "Can I WORK for you?" "Will you MARRY me?"

People will often say, "Yes!" Other people aren't mind readers. Often, they will happily agree to your request if they KNOW what you want.

USA Today recently ran a report on people who asked for a raise in salary. The study showed that 45% of women and 59% of men got more money when they asked for it. It's worth asking!

If you never ask – if you suffer in silence, if you always act the martyr and allow yourself to go without – your stomach keeps count. Asking for what you want keeps you happier and healthier.

IN A NUTSHELL
If you ask for it, you just might get it!

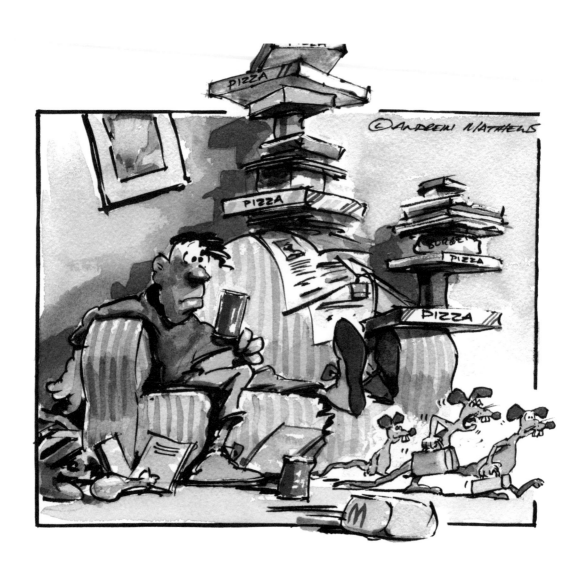

Throw out the Junk!

I know a lady called Nancy who has just bought a beautiful new Honda. But Nancy's garage is so full of bottles, old newspapers, cardboard boxes and other useless junk that she has to park her forty thousand dollar car in the street.

Living with junk affects your quality of life!

Psychological tests show that people suffer more stress in cluttered houses and cluttered offices. In clean spaces we feel more relaxed and energetic.

This must be one reason why people love to go camping – it's such a relief to wake up in the morning and not be surrounded by piles of old clothes and magazines and souvenirs from the last 21 family vacations.

Healthy rivers flush themselves out. Trees drop old leaves and fruit.

Your body feels better when you clean it out. So does your house.

A few thoughts on cleaning out:

1. Your old clothes will never come back into fashion! By the time bell-bottoms are back in vogue, the fabrics are different or the colours have changed. Designers aren't stupid – they know what you've got in your attic!

2. Sometimes we are reluctant to get rid of stuff because it would be admitting that we made a dumb decision to buy it in the first place. Relax! We all make silly purchases – so give it away!

3. Set small goals. Rather than say, "I'm going to clean the whole house", aim to do one cupboard. Then tackle another cupboard. Build momentum.

4. The hardest bit is starting. Once you've started, it's usually fun!

IN A NUTSHELL

Your life is an energy system. When you throw out things you create a vacuum, and you get things moving. Notice how often new things come along to replace what you give away.

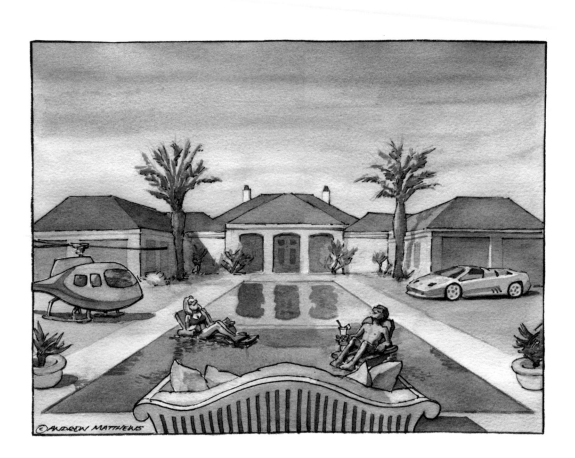

Prosperity

Some people seem to get respect wherever they go – whether they are in a department store or at the doctor's or in a hotel lobby.

What's their secret?
They treat themselves well – and other people follow.
People respect you when you respect you.

To quote my wife, Julie, "Everything affects everything else.
The way you walk affects the way you talk.
The way you dress affects the way you feel.
Respect yourself and you will be respected by others."

How can you feel like a mover and shaker when you have holes in your underwear – or when your toes are poking out of your socks?

It costs so little to keep a clean office or car.

Your home may not be grand but it can be tidy!

Where you live affects the way you feel. Create a space that will uplift you when you walk in the front door. Neatness costs nothing. Better to live in a one-room apartment that is clean, than in a mansion that's a mess.

A fellow asked Julie, "How can I possibly improve my apartment? All I can spare is $20."
Julie said, "Buy a broom!"

Fred says: "When I get successful, I'll quit living like a rat!" Wrong!
To be a success you have to begin to live it. You have to feel it now.

IN A NUTSHELL
People treat you as you treat you.

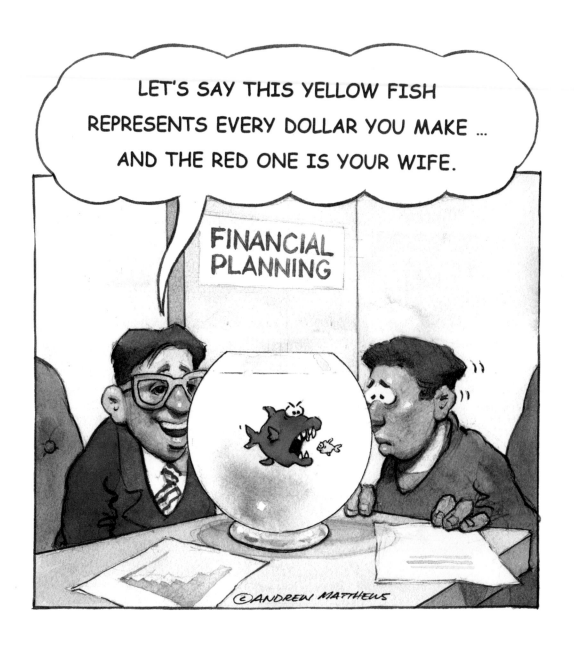

Save First!

Does this ever happen at your house ...
Your family sits down to eat a big apple pie – and in minutes, the whole pie disappears!
Even when no one is hungry, everybody eats!
Why? Because the pie is on the table.

Does this ever happen at your house ...
You get your pay cheque – and in no time, the whole thing disappears!
Even when you don't really need to spend it, you spend it.
Why? Because the money is there.

Now, back to that apple pie ...
If you want to save pie for tomorrow, anybody knows,
you don't put it all on the table.
You FIRST put a slice in the refrigerator - out of reach.

So how do you save cash for the future? You don't put it all in your wallet. You FIRST put a slice in a special bank account – out of reach.

Just a simple strategy ...
1. Open an account.
2. Every week, before you spend one cent, deposit 10%, automatically.

Soon you won't even miss that 10%.

You say, "But I earn so little!" Then just save a little! It will add up.

Lots of people can make big money.
Few people can save big money!

You say, "When I start making big dollars, then I'll save!"
You probably won't!
Better make it a habit now!

IN A NUTSHELL

Here's the difference between rich and poor:
Poor people spend first and save what is left.
Rich people save first and spend what is left.

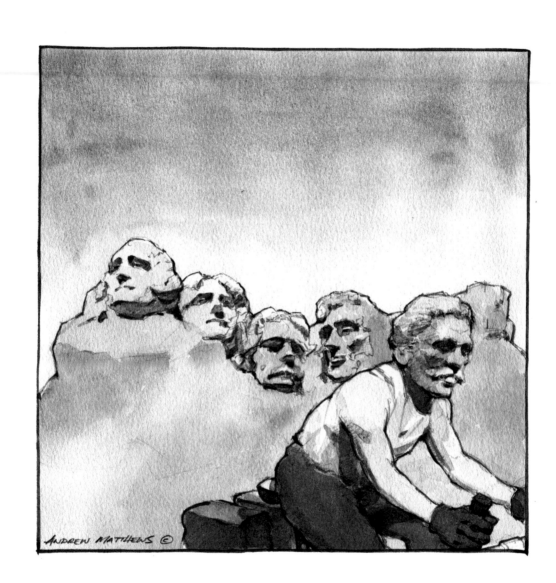

Just do it!

Recently my friend Colin Martin hopped on a bicycle and rode across North America. Vancouver to New York, 7136 kilometres ... just for the fun of it.

He had plenty of excuses NOT to do it:
   a) It wasn't cheap. He had to fly to America. He had to quit work for 2 months.
   b) It wasn't convenient. He has three young children.
   c) He was 53.

But Colin says: "No time is a perfect time. If you really want to do something, you have to put the time aside, and then just do it."

AN INTERESTING LIFE DOESN'T JUST HAPPEN TO YOU. You choose it. You plan it.

Peter Manuel is the principal at my old school, Victor Harbor High. Aged 18, Peter decided to learn a new skill each year of his life.

He is now 62. He has learned carpentry, pottery, tried drama, painted watercolours, learned some German, studied plastics, learned how to lay bricks ...

Says Peter: "That decision changed my life. At some things, like piano, I was terrible - but I had fun trying!"

If there is something you really want to do, no time will ever be perfect.

IN A NUTSHELL

What do you really want to do?
What will you do today to make it happen?

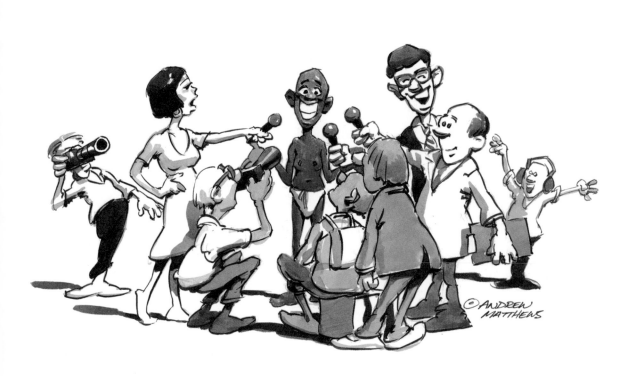

Your Best

Eric Moussambani swam for Equatorial Guinea at the 2000 Olympics. He didn't win.

Eric had never seen a big swimming pool before.
At home he trains in a 20 metre pool – in a hotel!

The two other entrants in his heat – from Niger and Tajikistan – were both disqualified for false starts, so Eric had to swim by himself.

Also, Eric had never swum a 100 metre race before – something the crowd soon suspected. He swam with his head out of the water and he barely kicked his legs.

In the first lap he was really struggling.

In the second lap he was nearly drowning.

But Eric gave it everything he had.

Thirty metres from the finish, 17,000 spectators began to cheer him home, and with each stroke the roar got louder. Ten metres out, he was bobbing like a cork but the crowd was going bananas.

When Moussambani finally hit the wall, the cheering and stamping all but lifted the roof off the stadium.

His time of 1 minute 52 seconds was about a minute slower than all the other competitors.

Who cared? Eric Moussambani had given his all.

IN A NUTSHELL

When people know you have given your very best, they usually support you.

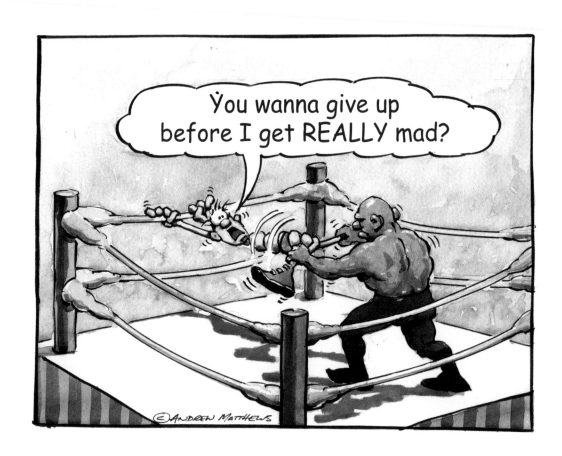

When to Quit?

Imagine you've started learning piano – and already you are thinking: "This is too hard. Maybe I'll learn the triangle ..."

Or imagine you've begun selling real estate. And you can't believe how many deals collapse!

You ask yourself, "Is it time to quit and look for something easier?"

The best time to quit is AFTER YOU'VE SUCCEEDED!

Why? Because success is more about persistence than talent. With practice you can probably do most things quite well – maybe not like an expert, but reasonably well. And you don't know how much fun something is until you can do it reasonably well.

Until you can play a dozen songs on your piano, you'll never know the thrill of making music.

Until you have sold maybe twenty properties, you'll never know if it's more fun being a successful agent than being a starving agent.

Hang in there long enough to reach a target. Then decide if you'll quit.

It's like pizza. Until you've tasted good pizza, how do you know if you like pizza?

Of course, sometimes you try something and it's obvious, "This was a really dumb idea!" But otherwise, it's all about persistence.

When you finish whatever you start, two things happen:
1. You consider carefully before starting something, and
2. You develop a success habit.

IN A NUTSHELL

Set a fair target, achieve it, and then decide if you'll quit.
It's amazing how a little success can change your mind!

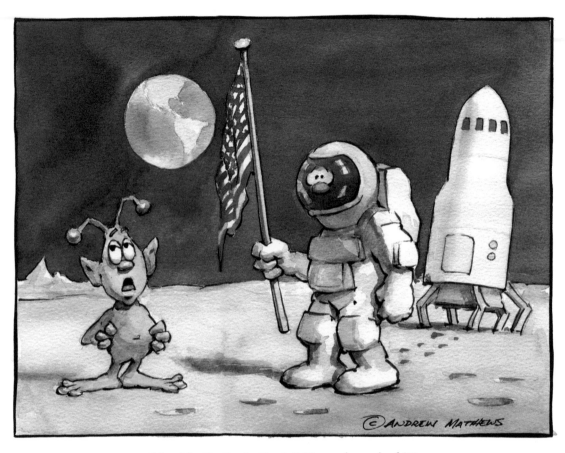

"A - M - E - R - I - C - A ? Never heard of it!
We did have a couple of fellas here from Amway ... "

What We Have

Imagine that we discovered life on Mars – even if it was only a tiny bug, or an ant with one leg ...

The world would go crazy! Splashed across the front page of every newspaper would be headlines, "THERE'S LIFE OUT THERE!"

Scientists would be ecstatic, "Another species!"

Now here's what's strange ... twenty-seven thousand of the earth's species of birds, plants, animals and insects became extinct last year.

That story never made the headlines.

Our tigers and pandas and frogs are disappearing. Meanwhile, we look for signs of life in outer space!

How often do we overlook the great things we have – and go looking for new stuff?

We do the same thing in relationships!

When we finally realise what we had, it's gone.

IN A NUTSHELL

The first trick to happiness – and success – is to appreciate what we've already got.

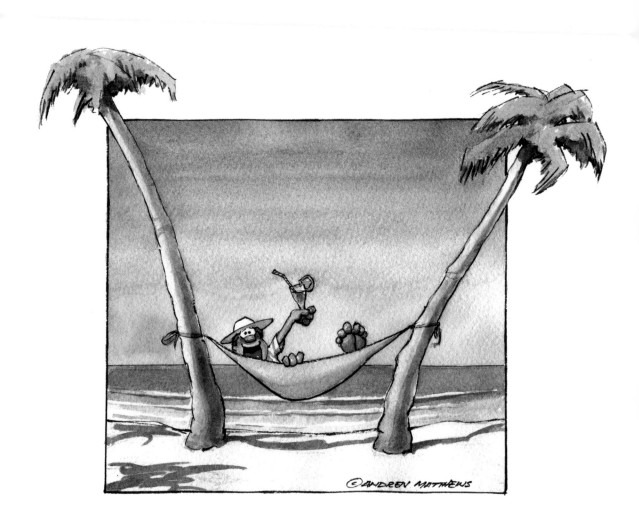

Everything Is Connected!

Have you noticed that whenever you exercise regularly, you feel like eating healthier food?

Have you noticed that when you eat healthier food, you have more energy – so you feel like exercising more?

Everything in life is connected.

Effort you put into one part of your life affects all the other parts.

When you are happy at home, you are happier at work.

When you are happy at work, you are happier at home.

So what does all this mean?

1. That to improve your life you can start on ANY positive path.
   You might start with a savings plan, a goal list, a fitness program or a commitment to spend more time with your children. That positive path will lead to other positive results because everything is connected.

2. It doesn't matter WHERE you start to put more effort into your life. It matters THAT you start.

3. It works both ways! If you let one part of your life collapse, everything will begin to spiral downward. This keeps us paying attention!

IN A NUTSHELL

Everything you do matters!
Happiness is a daily decision.

Sebastian's Story

Dear Mr Matthews,

I first read your book two years ago when my life was at a point of disaster. I was taking drugs, cheating on girlfriends, stealing and just constantly feeling depressed.

After reading your book I somehow turned my life around completely. I've stopped taking drugs, I've had a girlfriend for almost two years and we've worked together to get a very nice home filled with nice furniture, a car and even our pet budgie "Cosmo".

Last year I returned to school and did my two final years of high school, crammed into one. I'm currently studying financial planning at university.

Two years ago I was a drugged up loser with nothing to my name but debt. Now I am heading in the right direction with a much better standard of life.

Your book has literally changed my life around. I use FOLLOW YOUR HEART as a reference whenever I have a problem in my life. You are my favourite author. To me your book is my modern day Bible.

Yours faithfully
Sebastian Bruce
Brisbane, Queensland

Dear Mr. Matthews,

Thank you very, very much for the books you wrote!

I "found" your books about five years ago, when I was in a desperate situation: father had a heart attack, my husband a bad accident, Mum diagnosed with carcinoma, and to complete the disaster, I lost my job - all within 3 months!

Reading your books was like a helping hand. One moment I was drowning and then I suddenly felt safe.

Thank you so very much!

Kindest regards
Rosanna Monaco
Zurich, Switzerland

Dear Andrew,

Over the past 12 months I've been on a spiritual journey traveling and reading about life. You have had a huge impact on my success and happiness.

Call me a "happiness junkie" but I was looking forward to getting home to listen to your audio program 144 STRATEGIES for SUCCESS and HAPPINESS.

Whilst the anticipation of the CDs goes against the Bhuddist principles of attachment, I had to make an exception.

I was so engrossed in listening and loved every second. Thanks for providing me with guidance yet again.

Stephen Leong
Sydney, Australia

Nancy's Story

Dear Andrew:

I grew up in an alcoholic family and suffered many years from guilt and low self-esteem.

Before I was introduced to your books I relied on other people and things to make me happy. I went through bouts of alcohol and drug use, I went to therapy and had to take anti-depressants.

Now, having read your books over three years ago, I have realized I do deserve happiness and success, and I am experiencing it for the first time.

I listen to your CDs 144 STRATEGIES for SUCCESS and HAPPINESS every night before I go to bed. I have gained confidence in my self and confidence in my work.

My boss noticed my new found confidence and improved self esteem and I have received two promotions. I recently received an award from the bank that I work for for "Excellence in Service". I also received a $2500 bonus from the board of directors along with a letter praising me on my job performance and loyalty.

Today I am HAPPY to say I am confident, successful, prosperous and alcohol and drug free!

Again thank you and bless you.

Nancy Hayes
Tok, Alaska, USA